"Transformative Wellness: A Comprehensive Guide to Health, Fitness, Beauty, and Diet Mastery"

BY

Mollah Morshed

Chapters:

In a world where the pursuit of well-being takes center stage, "Transformative Wellness: A Comprehensive Guide to Health, Fitness, Beauty, and Diet Mastery" emerges as a beacon of enlightenment. This book is not just a guide; it is a roadmap to a holistic lifestyle that integrates health, fitness, beauty, and diet into a transformative journey towards overall wellness.

Chapter 1:

Introduction to Transformative Wellness

- Setting the foundation for holistic well-being

Understanding Holistic Wellness:

Embark on a journey that goes beyond conventional health approaches. Holistic well-being encompasses the integration of physical, mental, and emotional health. This chapter lays the groundwork for embracing a comprehensive view of wellness.

Understanding Holistic Wellness: Nurturing Balance in Mind, Body, and Spirit

Holistic wellness is a comprehensive approach to health that recognizes the interconnectedness of various facets of an individual's life. It goes beyond the traditional focus on physical health and includes mental, emotional, social, and even spiritual well-being. This holistic perspective views a person as a whole, understanding that each aspect of their life contributes to their overall state of wellness. Let's explore the key components and principles that form the foundation of holistic wellness:

1. Mind-Body Connection:

Holistic wellness acknowledges the intricate connection between the mind and the body. Mental and emotional well-being significantly impact physical health, and vice versa. For example, chronic stress or unresolved emotional issues can manifest in physical symptoms, highlighting the importance of addressing mental and emotional aspects for holistic health. Practices such as mindfulness, meditation, and cognitive-behavioral techniques bridge the gap between mental and physical well-being.

2. Emotional Wellness:

Emotional wellness involves recognizing, understanding, and managing one's emotions in a healthy way. It's about cultivating resilience, coping with stress, and fostering positive relationships. Emotional well-being contributes to overall life satisfaction and influences decision-making, communication, and the ability to navigate life's challenges. Practices like self-reflection, therapy, and mindfulness can enhance emotional wellness.

3. Social Well-Being:

Human beings are inherently social creatures, and social connections play a pivotal role in holistic wellness. Building and maintaining positive relationships contribute to a sense of belonging, support, and fulfillment. Social well-being involves effective communication, empathy, and the ability to create and sustain meaningful connections. Engaging in social activities, spending time with loved ones, and participating in community events are integral components of holistic wellness.

4. Physical Health:

While holistic wellness extends beyond physical health, it still recognizes the importance of taking care of the body. This involves regular exercise, a balanced and nutritious diet, sufficient sleep, and preventive healthcare measures. Physical health is not seen in isolation but as part of the broader context of well-being. Exercise, for instance, is not only beneficial for physical fitness but also plays a role in reducing stress and improving mood.

5. Intellectual Wellness:

Intellectual wellness involves the pursuit of knowledge, creativity, and continuous learning. Engaging in intellectually stimulating activities, seeking new experiences, and challenging oneself mentally contribute to a sense of intellectual well-being. This can involve pursuing hobbies, reading, attending educational events, or participating in activities that stimulate cognitive function.

6. Environmental Well-Being:

Holistic wellness also considers the impact of the environment on an individual's health. This includes the physical surroundings, workplace, and broader community. A clean and safe environment, access to nature, and sustainable practices contribute to environmental well-being. Creating a living and working space that aligns with one's values enhances the overall sense of wellness.

7. Spiritual Wellness:

Spiritual wellness does not necessarily relate to religious beliefs but encompasses a sense of purpose, meaning, and connection to something greater than oneself. It involves exploring one's values, beliefs, and the quest for inner peace. Practices such as meditation, mindfulness, and spending time in nature can foster spiritual well-being. It's about aligning one's actions with a sense of purpose and finding meaning in life.

8. Holistic Nutrition:

Holistic wellness places importance on nutrition as a fundamental aspect of well-being. It involves nourishing the body with whole, nutrient-dense foods and recognizing the relationship between diet and overall health. Holistic nutrition considers individual needs, food sensitivities, and the role of food in promoting not only physical health but also emotional and mental well-being.

9. Holistic Approaches to Healing:

Holistic wellness embraces alternative and complementary approaches to healing, viewing the body's natural ability to heal itself when supported in various ways. This might include practices such as acupuncture, chiropractic care, herbal medicine, or energy healing. These modalities focus on addressing imbalances in the body, mind, and spirit to promote overall well-being.

10. Holistic Stress Management:

Stress is an inevitable part of life, and holistic wellness emphasizes effective stress management strategies. This involves not only addressing the external stressors but also cultivating resilience from within. Mind-body practices, relaxation techniques, and time spent in activities that bring joy contribute to holistic stress management.

11. Mindful Living:

Holistic wellness encourages mindful living, which involves being fully present in the current moment. Mindfulness practices help individuals become more aware of their thoughts, emotions, and physical sensations. This heightened awareness fosters a deeper connection with oneself and the surrounding environment, contributing to overall well-being.

12. Preventive Healthcare:

Rather than waiting for illness to manifest, holistic wellness emphasizes preventive healthcare measures. This involves regular check-ups, screenings, and adopting a proactive approach to maintaining health. Preventive healthcare aligns with the philosophy of addressing potential issues before they become more significant challenges.

13. Work-Life Balance:

Achieving a balance between work and personal life is crucial for holistic wellness. This involves setting boundaries, prioritizing self-care, and recognizing the importance of downtime. A healthy work-life balance contributes to reduced stress, improved relationships, and enhanced overall well-being.

14. Holistic Self-Care Practices:

Self-care is a cornerstone of holistic wellness, involving intentional practices that nurture the mind, body, and spirit. This might include activities such as journaling, taking baths, practicing gratitude, or engaging in hobbies. Holistic self-care is not just about pampering oneself but aligning with practices that contribute to overall well-being.

15. Personal Responsibility and Empowerment:

Holistic wellness places a significant emphasis on personal responsibility and empowerment. It encourages individuals to take an active role in their health and well-being. This involves making informed choices, advocating for oneself in healthcare decisions, and recognizing the impact of lifestyle choices on overall wellness.

In essence, understanding holistic wellness is about recognizing the interplay between various aspects of life and taking a proactive and integrated approach to health. It's a philosophy that goes beyond treating symptoms and aims to create a balanced and fulfilling life. By embracing holistic wellness, individuals can foster resilience, cultivate a positive outlook, and navigate life's challenges with a sense of purpose and vitality.

The Interconnectedness of Health, Fitness, Beauty, and Diet:

Discover how these pillars of transformative wellness are interconnected. A balanced approach to health involves harmonizing fitness routines, dietary choices, and beauty practices to create a synergy that propels you toward a more fulfilling and vibrant life.

Setting the Foundation for Holistic Well-being

Mind-Body Connection:

Explore the profound connection between the mind and body. Learn how thoughts, emotions, and mental well-being play a pivotal role in shaping physical health. Uncover practices that promote a positive mindset as the cornerstone of transformative wellness.

The Power of Prevention:

Dive into the importance of preventive health measures. Understand how proactively managing your health through lifestyle choices can prevent illnesses and lay the foundation for a resilient and thriving body.

Holistic Nutrition Basics:

Get acquainted with the principles of holistic nutrition. This section provides insights into the nourishment your body needs for optimal function, energy, and longevity. Learn to view food not just as sustenance but as a source of vitality.

Balancing Act: Finding Harmony in Life's Demands:

Modern life can be demanding, but achieving transformative wellness requires balance. Explore strategies for harmonizing work, relationships, and personal time to ensure that your pursuit of well-being enhances every aspect of your life.

Embarking on Your Transformative Journey

Assessing Your Current Wellness Status:

Before embarking on any journey, it's essential to know where you stand. Utilize self-assessment tools and reflective exercises to gauge your current well-being status. This chapter provides a roadmap for setting personalized goals.

Defining Your Vision of Wellness:

What does wellness mean to you? Clarify your vision and goals for transformative wellness. Understand that it's a unique and personal journey, and your aspirations will guide your path toward a healthier, more vibrant you.

Conclusion: Your Invitation to Transformation

As we conclude the first chapter of "Transformative Wellness," you stand at the threshold of a transformative journey. Armed with knowledge, inspiration, and practical insights, you are ready to take charge of your holistic well-being. This chapter serves as the foundation, the first step towards a life where health, fitness, beauty, and diet converge to create a symphony of transformative wellness.

In the upcoming chapters, we'll delve deeper into each aspect, offering actionable steps, expert advice, and a wealth of information to empower you on your quest for mastery in health, fitness, beauty, and diet. Are you ready to transform your life? The journey begins here.

Chapter:2

Understanding the Fundamentals of Health**

- Exploring the key principles of physical and mental well-being

Understanding the Fundamentals of Health

In the intricate tapestry of human existence, health emerges as the foundational thread that weaves together the fabric of our lives. It encompasses not only the absence of disease but also the harmonious interplay between physical and mental well-being. This chapter embarks on a journey to explore the key principles of health, unraveling the intricacies that define a balanced and flourishing life.

1.1 The Holistic Nature of Health

Health is not a mere absence of illness; it is a state of complete physical, mental, and social well-being. This holistic perspective, as defined by the World Health Organization, acknowledges the interconnectedness of various facets of our lives. Physical health, mental stability, and social harmony form an inseparable trinity, each influencing and nurturing the others.

1.1.1 Physical Well-being

At the core of our existence lies the temple of the body, a miraculous vessel that demands care and respect. Physical well-being is the foundation upon which a robust and healthy life is built. This encompasses aspects such as nutrition, exercise, sleep, and the avoidance of harmful substances.

Nutrition: A balanced diet is the cornerstone of physical health. Nutrient-rich foods provide the essential vitamins, minerals, and energy needed for the body to function optimally. Understanding the importance of a diverse and well-rounded diet empowers individuals to make informed choices about their nutrition.

Exercise: The human body is designed for movement, and regular exercise is pivotal for maintaining optimal health. It not only strengthens muscles and bones but also contributes to cardiovascular health, mental well-being, and overall vitality. Exploring different forms of physical activity allows individuals to find joy in movement, transforming exercise from a routine into a lifestyle.

Sleep: The restorative power of sleep cannot be overstated. During this seemingly passive state, the body undergoes crucial processes of repair and rejuvenation. Understanding the significance of quality sleep and adopting healthy sleep hygiene practices promotes physical vitality and mental clarity.

Substance Avoidance: Harmful substances, such as tobacco and excessive alcohol, pose significant threats to physical health. An awareness of the detrimental effects of these substances empowers individuals to make choices that prioritize long-term well-being over momentary pleasure.

1.1.2 Mental Well-being

The mind, a realm of infinite complexity, plays a paramount role in shaping our experiences and perceptions. Mental well-being involves achieving a state of balance, resilience, and emotional intelligence.

Emotional Resilience: Life is a journey filled with both triumphs and tribulations. Developing emotional resilience equips individuals with the ability to navigate challenges, bounce back from setbacks, and cultivate a positive outlook. Techniques such as mindfulness and stress management become invaluable tools in fostering emotional well-being.

Social Connections: Humans are inherently social beings, and the quality of our social connections profoundly impacts mental health. Building and maintaining positive relationships provide a support system that fosters emotional well-being. Understanding the importance of communication, empathy, and connection cultivates a sense of belonging and purpose.

Mind-Body Connection: The intricate dance between the mind and body is a testament to their inseparable nature. Practices such as meditation, yoga, and deep breathing exercises underscore the profound impact of mental well-being on physical health. Cultivating an awareness of this mind-body connection opens avenues for holistic health promotion.

1.2 The Interplay of Physical and Mental Well-being

The boundaries between physical and mental health are fluid, with each influencing and shaping the other. Recognizing this symbiotic relationship is essential for crafting a comprehensive approach to well-being.

1.2.1 Stress and Its Impact

Stress, a ubiquitous companion in modern life, serves as a poignant example of the interconnectedness of physical and mental health. While stressors may originate from external factors, the physiological response to stress has profound implications for overall well-being.

Hormonal Response: When faced with stress, the body initiates a cascade of hormonal responses, including the release of cortisol and adrenaline. While these responses are adaptive in the short term, chronic exposure to stress hormones can lead to a range of physical ailments, from cardiovascular issues to compromised immune function.

Psychological Impact: On the mental front, chronic stress can contribute to anxiety, depression, and other mental health disorders. Understanding the dual impact of stress underscores the importance of adopting coping mechanisms that address both the physical and psychological aspects of well-being.

1.2.2 The Gut-Brain Axis

The gut, often referred to as the "second brain," exemplifies the intricate connection between physical and mental health. The gut-brain axis, a bidirectional communication system, highlights how the health of the digestive system can influence mental well-being and vice versa.

Microbiome Influence: The gut microbiome, a diverse community of microorganisms residing in the digestive tract, plays a pivotal role in digestion, nutrient absorption, and immune function. Emerging research suggests that the microbiome also exerts a significant influence on mental health, with alterations in gut flora linked to conditions such as depression and anxiety.

Nutrient Absorption: A healthy gut is essential for the efficient absorption of nutrients that support brain function. Conversely, poor mental health can manifest in digestive issues, emphasizing the interconnectedness of these two systems.

1.3 Navigating the Landscape of Preventive Health

Preventive health measures form the bedrock of a proactive and sustainable approach to well-being. Understanding the fundamentals of preventive health empowers individuals to take charge of their health destinies.

1.3.1 Screening and Early Detection

Regular health screenings serve as a preemptive strike against potential health threats. From routine blood tests to cancer screenings, early detection allows for timely intervention and management. Understanding the importance of regular check-ups fosters a culture of proactive health care.

1.3.2 Vaccinations and Immunizations

In the realm of infectious diseases, vaccinations stand as formidable guardians of public health. Understanding the role of vaccines in preventing diseases not only safeguards individual well-being but also contributes to community immunity. Navigating through misinformation and embracing evidence-based vaccination practices is essential for the collective health of societies.

1.3.3 Lifestyle Modification

The choices we make in our daily lives wield significant influence over our health trajectories. Adopting a proactive stance toward well-being involves conscious lifestyle modifications.

Dietary Choices: The adage "you are what you eat" encapsulates the profound impact of dietary choices on health. Understanding the principles of nutrition empowers individuals to make informed decisions that nourish the body and mind.

Physical Activity: The sedentary nature of modern lifestyles poses a threat to physical health. Incorporating regular physical activity into daily routines is a fundamental step toward preventing a myriad of health conditions. Understanding the diverse options for exercise allows individuals to find activities that resonate with their preferences and lifestyles.

Stress Management: Recognizing the inevitability of stress in life prompts a proactive approach to stress management. Techniques such as meditation, yoga, and mindfulness offer effective tools for mitigating the impact of stress on both physical and mental well-being.

1.4 Cultivating a Mindset of Health Literacy

Health literacy, the ability to obtain, understand, and apply health information, is a cornerstone for making informed decisions about one's well-being. Navigating the labyrinth of health information requires a discerning mindset and a commitment to continuous learning.

Chapter 3:
The Science of Fitness
- Unraveling the Mysteries of Effective Workout
Routines and Exercises

Introduction

In the pursuit of optimal health and well-being, few aspects are as crucial as physical fitness. The human body is a complex and adaptive system, and understanding the science behind effective workout routines and exercises is key to unlocking its full potential. In this chapter, we delve into the intricacies of fitness science, exploring the principles that govern effective workouts and shedding light on the mysteries of exercise physiology.

1. The Physiology of Exercise

To comprehend the science of fitness, one must first grasp the underlying physiology of exercise. The human body responds to physical activity in intricate ways, involving various systems and processes. At its core, exercise induces a cascade of physiological responses aimed at maintaining homeostasis and adapting to the imposed demands.

1.1. The Cardiovascular System

A fundamental aspect of exercise physiology is the impact on the cardiovascular system. Regular exercise enhances cardiovascular health by strengthening the heart, improving blood circulation, and optimizing oxygen transport to tissues. Aerobic exercises, such as running or cycling, are particularly effective in promoting cardiovascular fitness, leading to benefits like reduced risk of heart disease and improved endurance.

1.2. Muscular System Adaptations

Resistance training, on the other hand, primarily targets the muscular system. Progressive resistance exercises induce microtrauma in muscle fibers, prompting the body to repair and strengthen them. This process, known as hypertrophy, results in increased muscle mass and strength. Understanding the principles of overload, progression, and specificity is crucial for designing effective resistance training programs.

1.3. Metabolic Responses to Exercise

Exercise also has profound effects on metabolism. High-intensity interval training (HIIT), for instance, has gained popularity for its ability to enhance metabolic rate and promote fat loss. The science behind this lies in the post-exercise oxygen consumption (EPOC), where the body continues to burn calories even after the workout, contributing to weight management.

2. Principles of Effective Workout Routines

With the physiological foundations in mind, constructing effective workout routines becomes a matter of applying key principles. These principles serve as guiding forces, ensuring that exercise programs are both safe and efficient in achieving desired outcomes.

2.1. Individualization

No two individuals are alike, and effective workout routines must be tailored to individual characteristics such as age, fitness level, and health status. Individualization extends beyond just exercise selection; it involves customizing intensity, volume, and frequency to align with personal goals and capacities.

2.2. Progressive Overload

The principle of progressive overload is central to the effectiveness of any workout routine. It entails gradually increasing the stress placed on the body to elicit continuous adaptations. This can be achieved by manipulating factors like weight, repetitions, sets, or intensity. Failing to incorporate progressive overload may lead to plateaus in performance and hinder long-term progress.

2.3. Specificity

The principle of specificity dictates that training adaptations are specific to the type of exercise performed. Tailoring workouts to align with specific goals ensures that the body adapts in the desired manner. For example, a marathon runner would focus on endurance training, while a powerlifter would prioritize strength training.

2.4. Rest and Recovery

Optimal results are not solely achieved through intense workouts; adequate rest and recovery are equally vital. Overtraining can lead to fatigue, decreased performance, and increased risk of injury. Understanding the balance between training and recovery is crucial for sustained progress.

3. The Role of Nutrition in Fitness

The science of fitness extends beyond the gym, encompassing the critical role of nutrition in supporting exercise and promoting overall well-being. Proper nutrition is the fuel that powers the body through workouts, aids in recovery, and facilitates the desired physiological adaptations.

3.1. Macronutrients and Micronutrients

A well-balanced diet provides the necessary macronutrients – carbohydrates, proteins, and fats – and micronutrients – vitamins and minerals – essential for optimal health and performance. Each macronutrient plays a unique role, with carbohydrates serving as the primary energy source, proteins supporting muscle repair and growth, and fats contributing to overall health.

3.2. Timing of Nutrient Intake

The timing of nutrient intake can significantly impact exercise performance and recovery. Consuming carbohydrates before workouts provides a readily available energy source, while post-workout protein intake supports muscle protein synthesis and repair. Proper hydration is equally crucial, as dehydration can impair physical performance and delay recovery.

3.3. Nutritional Strategies for Different Goals

Different fitness goals require specific nutritional strategies. For those aiming to build muscle, a slight caloric surplus and increased protein intake are essential. Conversely, individuals focused on weight loss should aim for a caloric deficit while maintaining adequate protein intake to preserve lean muscle mass. Understanding the nuanced relationship between nutrition and fitness goals is key to achieving desired outcomes.

4. The Psychology of Exercise Adherence

While understanding the physiological and nutritional aspects of fitness is essential, adherence to a workout routine often hinges on psychological factors. Motivation, goal-setting, and mindset play pivotal roles in sustaining long-term commitment to exercise.

4.1. Motivation and Goal-Setting

Motivation serves as the driving force behind consistent exercise. Identifying intrinsic and extrinsic motivators can help individuals stay committed to their fitness journey. Goal-setting, whether short-term or long-term, provides a roadmap for progress and fosters a sense of achievement.

4.2. Mind-Body Connection

The mind-body connection is a powerful aspect of fitness that goes beyond physical exertion. Practices such as mindfulness, meditation, and yoga can enhance the connection between mental and physical well-being, reducing stress and promoting overall resilience.

4.3. Social Support and Accountability

Engaging in fitness activities with others can provide a sense of community and accountability. Whether through group classes, workout partners, or online communities, social support can positively impact motivation and adherence.

5. Emerging Trends and Technologies in Fitness

The field of fitness is continuously evolving, with emerging trends and technologies reshaping the way individuals approach their workouts. From wearable fitness trackers to virtual reality workouts, these advancements offer new avenues for enhancing the effectiveness and enjoyment of exercise.

5.1. Wearable Technology

Wearable devices, such as fitness trackers and smartwatches, have become ubiquitous in the fitness landscape. These devices monitor metrics such as heart rate, steps taken, and calories burned, providing users with real-time feedback and insights into their physical activity. The integration of technology into fitness not only enhances data tracking but also fosters motivation through gamification and goal-setting features.

5.2. Virtual and Augmented Reality

Virtual and augmented reality technologies are revolutionizing the fitness experience. Virtual reality workouts transport users to immersive environments, making exercise more engaging and enjoyable. Augmented reality applications overlay digital information onto the real world, offering interactive and personalized workout experiences. These technologies have the potential to break down barriers to exercise adherence by providing variety and novelty in routines.

5.3. Artificial Intelligence in Personalized Fitness

Artificial intelligence (AI) is increasingly being utilized to personalize fitness routines. AI algorithms analyze individual data, including workout history, preferences, and physiological responses, to generate customized exercise programs. This level of personalization ensures that workouts align with individual goals and capabilities, maximizing effectiveness.

6. Challenges and Considerations in Fitness Science

As we unravel the mysteries of fitness through science, it is essential to acknowledge the challenges and considerations that accompany this pursuit. From misinformation to individual variability, navigating the complexities of fitness science requires a discerning approach.

Chapter 4:
Nutrition Essentials for a Healthy Lifestyle
- Delving into the Importance of Balanced and
Nourishing Diets

Introduction

Nutrition is the cornerstone of a healthy lifestyle, influencing not only physical well-being but also mental and emotional health. A balanced and nourishing diet provides the body with the essential nutrients it needs for optimal functioning, energy production, and disease prevention. In this chapter, we explore the fundamental principles of nutrition, the components of a well-rounded diet, and the profound impact of food choices on overall health.

1. The Basics of Nutrition

To understand the essentials of nutrition, one must first grasp the basic components that constitute a healthy diet. Nutrition is the science of how the body utilizes nutrients from the foods we consume to sustain life and promote health. These essential nutrients can be broadly categorized into macronutrients and micronutrients.

1.1. Macronutrients

Macronutrients are nutrients that the body requires in relatively large quantities to support essential physiological functions. The three primary macronutrients are carbohydrates, proteins, and fats.

1.1.1. Carbohydrates

Carbohydrates are the body's main source of energy. They are broken down into glucose, which fuels the cells and supports various bodily functions. Whole grains, fruits, vegetables, and legumes are excellent sources of complex carbohydrates, providing sustained energy and essential nutrients.

1.1.2. Proteins

Proteins play a crucial role in building and repairing tissues, supporting immune function, and serving as enzymes and hormones.

Good sources of protein include lean meats, poultry, fish, eggs, dairy products, legumes, and plant-based sources such as tofu and quinoa.

1.1.3. Fats

Dietary fats are essential for energy storage, hormone production, and the absorption of fat-soluble vitamins (A, D, E, and K). Healthy fat sources include avocados, nuts, seeds, olive oil, and fatty fish like salmon. Balancing the intake of saturated and unsaturated fats is key to promoting cardiovascular health.

1.2. Micronutrients

Micronutrients are essential in smaller amounts but are equally vital for maintaining health. They include vitamins and minerals, each playing unique roles in various physiological processes.

1.2.1. Vitamins

Vitamins are organic compounds that support specific biochemical reactions in the body. They can be water-soluble (e.g., vitamin C, B vitamins) or fat-soluble (e.g., vitamins A, D, E, K). A diverse and balanced diet is crucial for obtaining an adequate spectrum of vitamins, as each serves a distinct function in promoting health.

1.2.2. Minerals

Minerals are inorganic elements that play essential roles in bone health, nerve function, fluid balance, and other physiological processes. Common minerals include calcium, iron, magnesium, potassium, and zinc. Obtaining a variety of foods from different food groups ensures an adequate intake of these essential minerals.

2. The Importance of Balanced and Nourishing Diets

A balanced and nourishing diet is essential for overall health and well-being. The foods we choose to consume impact various aspects of our physiological and psychological health, making nutrition a cornerstone of preventive medicine.

2.1. Energy Balance

Maintaining a healthy weight is closely tied to achieving an energy balance – the relationship between the calories consumed and expended. Consuming more calories than the body needs leads to weight gain, while a calorie deficit results in weight loss. A balanced diet provides the right mix of macronutrients and ensures that caloric intake aligns with individual energy needs.

2.2. Disease Prevention

Nutrition plays a crucial role in preventing chronic diseases. A diet rich in fruits, vegetables, whole grains, and lean proteins has been associated with a reduced risk of conditions such as heart disease, diabetes, and certain cancers. Additionally, adequate intake of essential nutrients supports immune function, reducing susceptibility to infections and illnesses.

2.3. Cognitive Function and Mental Health

The link between nutrition and cognitive function is increasingly recognized. Nutrient-rich diets, including omega-3 fatty acids, antioxidants, and vitamins, have been shown to support brain health and cognitive performance. Furthermore, emerging research suggests a connection between diet and mental health, with certain nutrients playing a role in mood regulation and the prevention of mental health disorders.

2.4. Gut Health

The health of the gut microbiome, a complex community of microorganisms in the digestive tract, is influenced by diet. A diverse and fiber-rich diet supports the growth of beneficial gut bacteria, contributing to digestive health and the prevention of gastrointestinal issues. Fermented foods, such as yogurt and kimchi, can further enhance the diversity of the microbiome.

3. Components of a Well-Rounded Diet

Achieving a well-rounded diet involves incorporating a variety of foods from different food groups to ensure a broad spectrum of nutrients. The Dietary Guidelines for Americans provide recommendations for a healthy diet, emphasizing key components for balanced nutrition.

3.1. Fruits and Vegetables

Fruits and vegetables are rich in vitamins, minerals, fiber, and antioxidants. They play a crucial role in supporting overall health and are associated with a reduced risk of chronic diseases. Aim to include a colorful variety of fruits and vegetables in daily meals to maximize nutrient intake.

3.2. Whole Grains

Whole grains, such as brown rice, quinoa, oats, and whole wheat, provide complex carbohydrates, fiber, and essential nutrients. Choosing whole grains over refined grains ensures a steady release of energy and supports digestive health.

3.3. Lean Proteins

Incorporating lean protein sources into the diet is essential for muscle maintenance, repair, and overall body function. Choose lean meats, poultry, fish, eggs, legumes, and plant-based protein sources to meet protein needs without excess saturated fat.

3.4. Healthy Fats

Healthy fats, including monounsaturated and polyunsaturated fats, are vital for heart health and overall well-being. Sources of healthy fats include avocados, nuts, seeds, olive oil, and fatty fish. Limit the intake of saturated and trans fats found in processed and fried foods.

3.5. Dairy or Dairy Alternatives

Dairy products or fortified dairy alternatives are important sources of calcium and vitamin D, essential for bone health. Choose low-fat or fat-free options to minimize saturated fat intake. For those with lactose intolerance or dairy allergies, alternatives such as almond milk, soy milk, or fortified plant-based alternatives can be suitable.

3.6. Hydration

Water is essential for various physiological functions, including temperature regulation, digestion, and nutrient transport. Staying adequately hydrated supports overall health. While water is the best choice for hydration, herbal teas and infused water can add variety to fluid intake.

4. Dietary Patterns and Approaches

In addition to individual food choices, dietary patterns and approaches have gained attention for their impact on health. Various eating styles, such as the Mediterranean diet, DASH (Dietary Approaches to Stop Hypertension) diet, and plant-based diets, have demonstrated positive effects on cardiovascular health, weight management, and disease prevention.

4.1. The Mediterranean Diet

The Mediterranean diet is characterized by an abundance of fruits and vegetables, whole grains, olive oil, nuts, and seeds, with moderate intake of fish, poultry, and dairy. This dietary pattern has been associated with reduced risks of heart disease, stroke, and certain cancers, emphasizing the importance of plant-based foods and healthy fats.

4

.2. Plant-Based Diets

Plant-based diets, which prioritize plant-derived foods while minimizing or excluding animal products, have gained popularity for their health benefits and environmental sustainability. Vegetarian and vegan diets can provide all essential nutrients when well-planned, emphasizing the importance of incorporating a variety of plant-based foods to meet nutritional needs.

4.3. Intermittent Fasting

Intermittent fasting involves cycles of eating and fasting, with various approaches such as time-restricted eating or alternate-day fasting. Some studies suggest that intermittent fasting may have benefits for weight management, metabolic health, and longevity. However, individual responses to fasting can vary, and it may not be suitable for everyone.

5. Nutritional Challenges and Considerations

While understanding the fundamentals of nutrition is crucial, navigating the complexities of individual dietary needs, cultural preferences, and potential challenges is equally important. Several factors can influence nutritional choices and pose challenges to maintaining a healthy diet.

5.1. Individual Variability

Individuals have unique nutritional needs based on factors such as age, gender, activity level, and underlying health conditions. What works for one person may not be suitable for another. Consulting with healthcare professionals, such as registered dietitians, can provide personalized guidance tailored to individual requirements.

5.2. Cultural and Dietary Preferences

Cultural and dietary preferences play a significant role in shaping eating habits. Recognizing and respecting cultural diversity is essential for promoting dietary patterns that align with both health recommendations and individual preferences. Adapting traditional dishes with healthier ingredients can be a sustainable approach to meeting cultural and health goals.

5.3. Accessibility and Affordability

Access to nutritious foods can be influenced by factors such as geographic location, socioeconomic status, and food availability. Food deserts, areas with limited access to fresh and healthy foods, can pose challenges to maintaining a balanced diet. Efforts to improve food accessibility and affordability are crucial for promoting equitable access to nutritious options.

5.4. Emotional and Social Factors

Emotional and social factors can significantly impact eating behaviors. Stress, emotional eating, and social influences may lead to unhealthy food choices. Developing mindfulness around eating habits, seeking support from friends and family, and finding alternative coping mechanisms for stress can contribute to a healthier relationship with food.

6. Practical Tips for Implementing a Healthy Diet

Implementing a healthy diet involves making practical and sustainable changes to eating habits. Small, gradual adjustments can lead to long-term improvements in overall nutrition. Consider the following tips for incorporating healthy eating into daily life:

6.1. Meal Planning and Preparation

Plan meals ahead of time and prepare ingredients in advance to make healthier choices more convenient. Batch cooking and meal prepping can save time during busy days and reduce reliance on less nutritious options.

6.2. Portion Control

Practice portion control by being mindful of serving sizes. Use smaller plates to avoid overeating and listen to hunger and fullness cues to maintain a healthy balance.

6.3. Mindful Eating

Eat with awareness, savoring each bite and paying attention to hunger and fullness signals. Avoid distractions such as screens or work while eating to promote mindful eating habits.

6.4. Read Food Labels

Familiarize yourself with food labels to understand the nutritional content of packaged foods. Look for whole, minimally processed foods and be mindful of added sugars, sodium, and unhealthy fats.

6.5. Stay Hydrated

Prioritize hydration by drinking an adequate amount of water throughout the day. Limit sugary drinks and opt for water, herbal teas, or infused water as healthier alternatives.

6.6. Listen to Your Body

Recognize and respond to your body's signals. Eat when hungry, and stop when satisfied. Avoid restrictive diets that may lead to unhealthy relationships with food.

7. Future Directions in Nutrition Science

As our understanding of nutrition continues to evolve, ongoing research and advancements in technology will shape the future of nutrition science. From personalized nutrition to the exploration of the gut-brain axis, several exciting areas hold promise for enhancing our knowledge of how food influences health.

7.1. Personalized Nutrition

Advancements in genetics, microbiome research, and data analytics are paving the way for personalized nutrition approaches. Tailoring dietary recommendations to an individual's unique genetic makeup, microbiome composition, and health goals holds the potential to optimize nutrition outcomes.

7.2. Nutrigenomics

Nutrigenomics is a field that explores how individual genetic variations influence responses to specific nutrients and dietary patterns. Understanding the interplay between genetics and nutrition can lead to personalized dietary recommendations that account for genetic predispositions to certain health conditions.

7.3. Microbiome Research

Research on the gut microbiome continues to uncover the intricate relationship between the trillions of microorganisms in the digestive tract and overall health. The gut microbiome influences nutrient absorption, immune function, and even mental health. Probiotics, prebiotics, and personalized dietary recommendations may emerge as strategies to support a healthy gut microbiome.

7.4. Brain-Body Connection

Exploring the intricate connection between the brain and body through nutrition is an emerging area of interest. The gut-brain axis, which involves bidirectional communication between the gut and the central nervous system, is being investigated for its implications in mental health, cognitive function, and mood regulation.

Conclusion

Nutrition is a dynamic and multifaceted aspect of our lives, influencing our health and well-being in profound ways. A balanced and nourishing diet is not only a fundamental component of preventive medicine but also a key factor in promoting physical, mental, and emotional resilience. As we continue to unravel the complexities of nutrition science, the importance of making informed and sustainable food choices becomes increasingly evident. By embracing a holistic approach to nutrition that considers individual needs, cultural preferences, and emerging research, we can cultivate a healthy lifestyle that supports longevity and vitality.

Chapter 5:

Mindful Eating Practices

 - Cultivating awareness and a positive relationship with food

Introduction

In a world dominated by fast-paced lifestyles, hectic schedules, and an abundance of processed foods, the concept of mindful eating has emerged as a beacon of balance and well-being. Mindful eating is not just about what you eat, but how you eat. It involves cultivating a heightened awareness of your eating habits, making conscious food choices, and developing a positive relationship with food. This chapter will delve into the principles and practices of mindful eating, exploring its origins, benefits, and practical strategies to incorporate mindfulness into your meals.

Section 1: Understanding Mindful Eating

Subsection 1.1: The Roots of Mindful Eating

Mindful eating finds its roots in mindfulness, an ancient practice rooted in Buddhism. The concept of mindfulness revolves around being present in the current moment, paying attention to thoughts and feelings without judgment. Thich Nhat Hanh, a Vietnamese Zen Buddhist monk, is often credited with bringing mindfulness to the West and popularizing its application to eating. Mindful eating borrows from these principles, urging individuals to bring mindfulness into their relationship with food.

Subsection 1.2: The Mind-Body Connection

Mindful eating emphasizes the mind-body connection, recognizing that our thoughts and emotions profoundly impact our eating habits. Often, people turn to food as a source of comfort or distraction, leading to mindless eating. By fostering awareness of these habits, mindful eating seeks to create a more harmonious relationship between the mind and body, encouraging individuals to eat in response to hunger rather than emotions.

Section 2: The Benefits of Mindful Eating

Subsection 2.1: Improved Digestion and Nutrient Absorption

One of the primary benefits of mindful eating is its positive impact on digestion. When we eat mindfully, we engage our senses, savoring the flavors and textures of each bite. This heightened awareness triggers the body's digestive processes, promoting better nutrient absorption and overall digestive health.

Subsection 2.2: Weight Management

Contrary to conventional dieting approaches, mindful eating doesn't focus on strict rules or calorie counting. Instead, it encourages listening to your body's hunger and fullness cues. Studies have shown that individuals who practice mindful eating are more likely to maintain a healthy weight and experience fewer struggles with weight management.

Subsection 2.3: Enhanced Emotional Well-being

Mindful eating extends beyond the physical aspects of nourishment; it also addresses the emotional relationship with food. By being present and attentive during meals, individuals can develop a healthier response to emotions, reducing the likelihood of emotional eating. This emotional resilience contributes to overall mental well-being.

Section 3: Practical Strategies for Mindful Eating

Subsection 3.1: Bringing Mindfulness to the Table

The practice of mindful eating begins with creating a mindful environment. This includes minimizing distractions, such as electronic devices or television, and dedicating time solely to the act of eating. By focusing on the sensory experience of each bite, individuals can appreciate the flavors, aromas, and textures of their food.

Subsection 3.2: Listening to Your Body

One of the core principles of mindful eating is attuning to the body's signals of hunger and fullness. Rather than eating on autopilot or adhering to external cues, individuals learn to trust their bodies. This involves recognizing subtle hunger cues and stopping when comfortably full, fostering a healthier and more intuitive approach to eating.

Subsection 3.3: Mindful Food Choices

Mindful eating involves making conscious choices about what and how you eat. This includes selecting whole, nutrient-dense foods that nourish the body. By paying attention to the quality of the food consumed, individuals can develop a deeper appreciation for the role of nutrition in overall well-being.

Section 4: Overcoming Challenges in Mindful Eating

Subsection 4.1: Breaking the Habit of Multitasking

In a fast-paced world, multitasking has become a norm, even during meals. Mindful eating challenges this habit by encouraging individuals to focus solely on the act of eating. Overcoming the urge to check emails, scroll through social media, or watch television while eating is a crucial step in cultivating mindfulness.

Subsection 4.2: Dealing with Emotional Eating

Emotional eating is a common challenge that mindful eating addresses. By developing an awareness of emotional triggers, individuals can respond to emotions in healthier ways, reducing the reliance on food for comfort. Mindful practices, such as deep breathing or meditation, can be incorporated to manage emotions without turning to food.

Subsection 4.3: Patience and Persistence

Like any transformative practice, adopting mindful eating requires patience and persistence. Breaking ingrained habits takes time, and setbacks are a natural part of the process. Encouraging individuals to approach mindful eating with a sense of self-compassion and understanding fosters a sustainable and positive relationship with food.

Mindful Eating in Daily Life

Section 1: Mindful Eating in Different Culinary Traditions

Subsection 1.1: Eastern Influences

Eastern culinary traditions, particularly those rooted in mindfulness practices, offer valuable insights into mindful eating. Practices such as mindful tea drinking in Japan or mindful consumption of prasad in Hinduism showcase the integration of mindfulness into daily meals.

Subsection 1.2: Western Perspectives

While mindfulness may have Eastern origins, its principles have found resonance in Western cultures as well. From the slow food movement to mindful eating workshops, the West has increasingly embraced the idea of savoring each bite and fostering a positive relationship with food.

Section 2: Mindful Eating and Nutrition

Subsection 2.1: Conscious Nutrition Choices

Mindful eating is not about strict dietary rules but rather about making conscious choices that align with your body's needs. This section explores how individuals can integrate mindful eating principles into their nutrition decisions, emphasizing balance, variety, and moderation.

Subsection 2.2: Mindful Eating and Special Diets

Whether following a specific diet for health reasons or personal beliefs, mindful eating can complement various dietary approaches. From vegetarianism to intuitive eating, the principles of mindfulness can enhance the overall experience and benefits of these dietary choices.

Section 3: Mindful Eating Beyond the Plate

Subsection 3.1: Mindful Cooking

The practice of mindful eating extends to the preparation of food. Mindful cooking involves engaging all the senses during the cooking process, appreciating the colors, smells, and textures of ingredients. This approach not only enhances the culinary experience but also promotes a deeper connection with the food being prepared.

Subsection 3.2: Mindful Eating in Social Settings

Eating is often a social activity, and mindful eating can be practiced in group settings. This section explores how individuals can maintain mindfulness when dining with others, fostering a positive and shared experience around food.

Chapter 3: Mindful Eating for Health and Wellness

Section 1: Mindful Eating and Mental Health

Subsection 1.1: Mindful Eating and Stress Reduction

Stress is a common trigger for unhealthy eating habits. Mindful eating provides a valuable tool for managing stress by redirecting attention to the present moment and promoting a more thoughtful response to stressors.

Subsection 1.2: Mindful Eating and Mindful Living

Mindful eating is part of a broader philosophy of mindful living. This section explores how incorporating mindfulness into various aspects of life, including eating,

can contribute to overall mental well-being.

Section 2: Mindful Eating for Specific Health Conditions

Subsection 2.1: Mindful Eating and Digestive Disorders

For individuals with digestive disorders, mindful eating can offer relief by promoting a more relaxed and attentive approach to meals. Techniques such as mindful chewing and savoring can be particularly beneficial for those with conditions like irritable bowel syndrome (IBS).

Subsection 2.2: Mindful Eating and Weight-related Health Issues

Mindful eating has shown promise in addressing weight-related health issues such as obesity and diabetes. This section explores how the practice can be tailored to support individuals in managing these conditions effectively.

Section 3: Mindful Eating in Fitness and Exercise

Subsection 3.1: Mindful Eating and Exercise Performance

Fueling the body for exercise is a crucial aspect of fitness. Mindful eating can enhance exercise performance by ensuring that individuals provide their bodies with the right nutrients at the right times, promoting energy balance and recovery.

Subsection 3.2: Mindful Eating and Body Image in Fitness Culture

In a culture often obsessed with body image, mindful eating encourages a more compassionate and realistic view of one's body. This section explores how adopting mindful eating practices can contribute to a healthier relationship with body image within the fitness community.

Mindful Eating for Sustainable Living

Section 1: Mindful Eating and Sustainability

Subsection 1.1: The Environmental Impact of Food Choices

The choices we make in our diets have far-reaching effects on the environment. This section explores how mindful eating can extend beyond personal well-being to include considerations for sustainability, such as choosing locally sourced and seasonally available foods.

Subsection 1.2: Mindful Eating and Food Waste Reduction

Mindful eating involves appreciating the value of food and being conscious of food waste. This section discusses how mindful eating practices can contribute to reducing food waste at the individual and societal levels.

Section 2: Mindful Eating and Ethical Food Choices

Subsection 2.1: Mindful Eating and Animal Welfare

For those who choose to include animal products in their diets, mindful eating can involve making ethical choices that prioritize the well-being of animals. This section explores how mindfulness can extend to considerations of humane and sustainable animal agriculture.

Subsection 2.2: Mindful Eating and Fair Trade Practices

Mindful eating is not only about what you eat but also about the ethical implications of your food choices. This section examines how individuals can practice mindful eating by supporting fair trade practices and ethical sourcing of food products.

Cultivating Mindful Eating Habits for a Lifetime

Section 1: Mindful Eating Across the Lifespan

Subsection 1.1: Mindful Eating for Children and Adolescents

Instilling mindful eating habits from a young age can set the foundation for a lifetime of healthy eating. This section explores age-appropriate strategies to introduce mindfulness to children and adolescents, promoting a positive relationship with food.

Subsection 1.2: Mindful Eating for Aging Adults

As individuals age, their nutritional needs may change. Mindful eating can be a valuable tool for aging adults to adapt to these changes, fostering a continued appreciation for the joy of eating and supporting overall well-being.

Section 2: Integrating Mindful Eating into Everyday Life

Subsection 2.1: Overcoming Challenges in Long-Term Practice

Maintaining mindful eating habits over the long term may pose challenges. This section offers practical tips for overcoming obstacles and integrating mindfulness seamlessly into daily life, ensuring that it becomes a sustainable and enduring practice.

Subsection 2.2: Mindful Eating as a Lifelong Journey

Mindful eating is not a destination but a journey. This section emphasizes the importance of viewing mindful eating as a lifelong practice, adapting to changing circumstances and continuously deepening one's relationship with food.

Conclusion

In conclusion, mindful eating is a transformative practice that goes beyond the act of consuming food. It is a holistic approach to nourishment, emphasizing the connection between the mind, body, and the food we eat. By cultivating awareness and fostering a positive relationship with food, individuals can not only enhance their physical health but also experience a profound shift in their overall well-being. Through the exploration of its principles, benefits, practical strategies, and diverse applications, this chapter aims to empower readers to embark on a journey of mindful eating, unlocking the potential for a healthier and more fulfilling life.

Chapter 6:

Unlocking the Secrets of Beauty from Within

- Connecting internal well-being to external radiance

Introduction

Beauty has been a subject of fascination and pursuit for centuries. From ancient civilizations to modern societies, individuals have sought ways to enhance and celebrate their physical appearance. However, in the relentless pursuit of external beauty, the significance of internal well-being is often overlooked. This essay aims to delve into the profound connection between internal well-being and external radiance, exploring how our physical appearance is intricately linked to our mental, emotional, and physical health.

Body and Mind: A Symbiotic Relationship

The human body is a complex and interconnected system, where each part influences the others. Our mental and emotional states, in particular, play a crucial role in shaping our external appearance. Stress, anxiety, and other negative emotions can manifest physically, affecting skin health, hair quality, and overall radiance. Conversely, a positive mindset, emotional balance, and mental well-being can contribute to a more vibrant and attractive outward appearance.

Understanding the Stress-Beauty Connection

Stress is an inevitable part of life, but its impact on our physical appearance is often underestimated. Chronic stress triggers the release of hormones like cortisol, which can lead to a variety of adverse effects on the skin, such as acne, inflammation, and premature aging. Exploring stress management techniques, such as mindfulness, meditation, and yoga, can not only improve mental well-being but also promote healthier skin and a more radiant complexion.

The Gut-Skin Axis: Nourishing Beauty from Within

The phrase "you are what you eat" takes on a new dimension when considering the connection between gut health and skin radiance. The gut-skin axis, a bidirectional relationship between the gastrointestinal system and the skin, highlights the profound impact of nutrition on external beauty. A diet rich in antioxidants, vitamins, and essential nutrients can promote clear skin, strong nails, and shiny hair. Exploring the role of nutrition in enhancing beauty from within opens up avenues for holistic beauty practices that go beyond external cosmetics.

Holistic Approaches to Beauty

The beauty industry often focuses on external fixes, offering an array of skincare products, makeup, and cosmetic procedures. While these can contribute to enhancing appearance temporarily, their effects may be superficial if not supported by a holistic approach. Exploring holistic beauty practices involves addressing internal factors such as nutrition, hydration, sleep, and stress management. Integrating these elements into a comprehensive beauty routine can lead to longer-lasting and more authentic radiance.

Embracing Self-Care for Lasting Beauty

Self-care is a fundamental aspect of unlocking the secrets of beauty from within. It encompasses a range of practices that prioritize mental, emotional, and physical well-being. Adequate sleep, regular exercise, and nurturing relationships contribute to a positive self-image and overall radiance. By prioritizing self-care, individuals can cultivate a sense of inner beauty that transcends societal standards and embraces uniqueness.

Mindful Beauty: The Power of Perception

The way we perceive ourselves profoundly influences our external appearance. The concept of mindful beauty emphasizes the importance of cultivating a positive self-image and embracing individuality. Exploring the impact of self-esteem, body positivity, and self-love on beauty reveals that true radiance comes from accepting and celebrating one's unique features. Mindful beauty practices encourage individuals to break free from societal beauty norms and redefine their standards of attractiveness.

The Role of Exercise in Enhancing Beauty

Physical activity is not only essential for overall health but also plays a significant role in enhancing external beauty. Exercise promotes circulation, which nourishes the skin and brings a natural glow. Additionally, regular physical activity contributes to weight management, muscle tone, and posture, all of which influence how we present ourselves to the world. Exploring the symbiotic relationship between exercise and beauty provides insights into the transformative power of an active lifestyle.

Unlocking the Potential of Sleep for Beauty

Sleep is often referred to as the body's natural beauty treatment. During sleep, the body undergoes crucial processes of repair, regeneration, and hormone regulation. Lack of sleep can lead to dark circles, dull skin, and accelerated aging. Exploring the connection between sleep and beauty highlights the importance of establishing healthy sleep patterns for maintaining youthful skin, vibrant eyes, and an overall radiant appearance.

The Psychological Impact of Beauty Standards

Societal beauty standards can have a profound impact on an individual's perception of their own beauty. Exploring the psychological aspects of beauty standards reveals the influence of media, culture, and peer pressure on shaping our ideals of attractiveness. Understanding the psychological impact of these standards is crucial for developing a healthy relationship with one's appearance and embracing a more inclusive definition of beauty.

Cultural Perspectives on Beauty

Beauty standards vary across cultures, reflecting diverse ideals of attractiveness. Exploring different cultural perspectives on beauty unveils the richness of individual expressions and challenges the notion of a universal standard. Embracing cultural diversity in beauty practices encourages a more inclusive and expansive understanding of what is considered beautiful. By appreciating and incorporating diverse beauty traditions, individuals can unlock a broader spectrum of beauty from within.

The Impact of Environmental Factors on Beauty

Environmental factors, such as pollution and exposure to ultraviolet (UV) radiation, can significantly influence external appearance. Exploring the effects of environmental stressors on the skin and hair underscores the importance of protective measures. Incorporating skincare routines that include antioxidants and SPF, as well as adopting sustainable practices, can contribute to preserving beauty in the face of environmental challenges.

Technological Advancements in Beauty

Advancements in technology have revolutionized the beauty industry, offering innovative solutions for skincare, cosmetic procedures, and personalized beauty routines. Exploring the intersection of technology and beauty reveals the potential for tailored approaches that consider individual needs and preferences. From augmented reality in makeup applications to personalized skincare based on genetic factors, technology opens up new frontiers for unlocking the secrets of beauty from within.

Conclusion

In conclusion, the pursuit of beauty is a multifaceted journey that goes beyond external appearances. Unlocking the secrets of beauty from within involves recognizing the interconnectedness of internal well-being with external radiance. By understanding the impact of stress, nutrition, self-care, and cultural influences on beauty, individuals can adopt holistic approaches that promote lasting and authentic radiance. Embracing diversity, challenging societal beauty norms, and incorporating technological advancements contribute to a more inclusive and personalized understanding of beauty. Ultimately, the journey towards unlocking the secrets of beauty from within is a transformative process that nurtures not only physical appearance but also mental, emotional, and spiritual well-being.

Chapter 7:

Skincare Rituals for a Glowing Complexion**

- Tailoring a skincare routine for healthy and radiant skin

Introduction

The pursuit of a glowing complexion has been a timeless endeavor, transcending cultures and epochs. As the largest organ of the human body, the skin requires dedicated care and attention to maintain its health and radiance. This essay aims to explore the intricacies of skincare rituals, focusing on the importance of tailoring a personalized routine for achieving and sustaining a glowing complexion. From understanding individual skin types to selecting the right products, adopting effective cleansing techniques, and considering lifestyle factors, a holistic approach to skincare rituals is crucial for promoting healthy and radiant skin.

Understanding Your Skin: The Foundation of a Tailored Routine

Before delving into the world of skincare rituals, it is essential to understand the unique characteristics of your skin. Skin types vary widely, from oily and acne-prone to dry and sensitive. Identifying your skin type lays the foundation for a tailored skincare routine that addresses specific needs and concerns. Additionally, factors such as age, genetics, and environmental influences contribute to the dynamic nature of the skin. By gaining insights into your skin's individual requirements, you can create a targeted and effective skincare regimen.

The Basics of Skincare: Cleansing, Toning, and Moisturizing

A fundamental skincare routine comprises three essential steps: cleansing, toning, and moisturizing. These basic steps form the core of any regimen and lay the groundwork for additional treatments and products.

1. **Cleansing:**

Cleansing is the initial step to remove impurities, makeup, and excess oil from the skin. Choosing a cleanser that suits your skin type is crucial. For oily skin, a foaming or gel cleanser helps control excess oil, while those with dry skin may benefit from a hydrating or cream-based cleanser. Double cleansing, incorporating an oil-based cleanser followed by a water-based one, is effective for thoroughly removing impurities.

2. **Toning:**

Toning helps balance the skin's pH, tightens pores, and prepares the skin for subsequent products. Toners come in various formulations, including hydrating, exfoliating, and soothing options. Selecting a toner that complements your skin type and concerns enhances the overall effectiveness of your skincare routine.

3. **Moisturizing:**

Moisturizing is essential for maintaining skin hydration and preventing moisture loss. Even individuals with oily skin benefit from a lightweight, oil-free moisturizer. For those with dry skin, a richer moisturizer with ingredients like hyaluronic acid and glycerin provides intensive hydration. Including a moisturizer in your routine contributes to a supple and well-nourished complexion.

Targeted Treatments: Serums, Masks, and Spot Treatments

Beyond the basic steps, incorporating targeted treatments addresses specific concerns and enhances the overall efficacy of a skincare routine.

1. **Serums:**

Serums are concentrated formulations designed to address specific skin issues, such as hyperpigmentation, fine lines, and dehydration. Including serums with active ingredients like vitamin C, retinol, or hyaluronic acid can target particular concerns and contribute to a more radiant complexion.

2. **Masks:**

Face masks provide a boost of nutrients and address various skincare concerns. Sheet masks, clay masks, and overnight masks offer different benefits, from hydration and brightening to pore refinement and exfoliation. Introducing masks into your routine provides a pampering and rejuvenating experience for the skin.

3. **Spot Treatments:**

Spot treatments are designed to target specific blemishes, acne, or dark spots. Ingredients like salicylic acid, benzoyl peroxide, or niacinamide can be included in spot treatments to address these concerns directly. Incorporating spot treatments as needed helps maintain a clear and even complexion.

Sun Protection: A Non-Negotiable Step

One of the most crucial aspects of skincare is sun protection. Sun exposure contributes to premature aging, hyperpigmentation, and an increased risk of skin cancer. Integrating a broad-spectrum sunscreen with an SPF of at least 30 into your daily routine is non-negotiable. Sunscreen safeguards the skin from harmful UV rays, preserving its health and preventing long-term damage.

Customizing Your Routine: The Importance of Individualization

While general skincare principles provide a foundation, the key to a truly effective routine lies in customization. Factors such as climate, lifestyle, and seasonal changes can impact the skin, necessitating adjustments to your skincare regimen.

1. **Climate Considerations:**

The climate in which you live plays a significant role in determining your skin's needs. In humid conditions, lightweight and oil-free products may be preferred, while drier climates may require richer moisturizers. Adapting your routine to seasonal changes ensures that your skin receives the necessary care year-round.

2. **Lifestyle Factors:**

Lifestyle choices, including diet, exercise, and sleep, profoundly influence the skin. A well-balanced diet rich in antioxidants, hydration, and adequate sleep contributes to a healthier complexion. Regular exercise promotes blood circulation, which enhances the skin's natural radiance. Taking lifestyle factors into account allows for a more comprehensive approach to skincare.

3. **Age-Appropriate Skincare:**

As the skin undergoes changes with age, adjusting your skincare routine accordingly is crucial. Younger individuals may focus on preventative measures, including sunscreen and antioxidants. As skin matures, incorporating products with anti-aging ingredients, such as peptides and retinoids, becomes more relevant.

Holistic Approaches: Nutrition, Hydration, and Stress Management

Skincare rituals extend beyond topical products to encompass holistic approaches that address internal factors affecting the skin.

1. **Nutrition:**

A well-balanced diet rich in vitamins, minerals, and antioxidants contributes to skin health. Foods high in omega-3 fatty acids, such as salmon and walnuts, promote hydration and elasticity. Antioxidant-rich fruits and vegetables protect the skin from free radical damage, supporting a radiant complexion.

2. **Hydration:**

Adequate hydration is vital for skin health. Drinking enough water helps maintain skin elasticity and suppleness. Additionally, using hydrating products, such as hyaluronic acid serums, contributes to a plump and dewy complexion.

3. **Stress Management:**

Stress has a profound impact on the skin, contributing to inflammation, breakouts, and premature aging. Incorporating stress management techniques, such as meditation, deep breathing, or yoga, promotes both mental well-being and skin health.

Sustainability in Skincare: Conscious Choices for the Environment and the Skin

An emerging aspect of skincare rituals involves conscious choices that consider environmental impact and sustainability. As consumers become more environmentally aware, selecting products with eco-friendly packaging, cruelty-free formulations, and ethically sourced ingredients aligns skincare practices with a broader commitment to environmental responsibility.

Conclusion

In conclusion, skincare rituals for a glowing complexion involve a thoughtful and personalized approach that goes beyond surface-level care. Tailoring a skincare routine based on individual skin type, concerns, and lifestyle factors is fundamental to achieving and maintaining healthy and radiant skin. From the basics of cleansing, toning, and moisturizing to incorporating targeted treatments, sun protection, and holistic approaches, a comprehensive skincare regimen encompasses a variety of practices. By understanding the unique needs of your skin and adopting a customized routine, you embark on a journey towards not only external beauty but also long-term skin health and vitality.

Chapter 8:

Fitness for Every Body Type

- Customizing workout plans based on individual needs and preferences

Introduction

The fitness journey is a highly individualized and dynamic process, shaped by factors such as body type, fitness goals, and personal preferences. While societal standards often perpetuate a narrow definition of the ideal body, the concept of "Fitness for Every Body Type" challenges this narrative. This essay explores the importance of customizing workout plans to accommodate diverse body types, emphasizing inclusivity, health, and personalization. By understanding the unique characteristics of different body types and tailoring exercise routines accordingly, individuals can embark on a fitness journey that not only aligns with their goals but also celebrates the diversity of human bodies.

Body Types and Their Significance in Fitness

Before delving into the customization of workout plans, it's essential to recognize the various body types that exist. The three primary body types, commonly known as somatotypes, are ectomorph, mesomorph, and endomorph. Each type comes with its own set of characteristics, influencing factors such as metabolism, muscle development, and fat distribution.

1. **Ectomorph:**

   - Characteristics: Slim and lean physique, difficulty gaining muscle or weight.

   - Exercise Focus: Emphasis on muscle building and strength training to promote lean muscle mass.

2. **Mesomorph:**

   - Characteristics: Naturally muscular and athletic build, easier muscle development.

   - Exercise Focus: A balanced approach, combining strength training and cardiovascular exercises for overall fitness.

3. **Endomorph:**

   - Characteristics: Rounded or softer physique, tendency to gain weight easily.

   - Exercise Focus: Priority on metabolic conditioning, combining cardiovascular exercises with strength training for fat loss.

Understanding individual body types lays the groundwork for creating workout plans that capitalize on inherent strengths, address specific challenges, and align with personal fitness objectives.

Customizing Workout Plans for Ectomorphs

Ectomorphs often face challenges in gaining muscle mass and weight. Customizing workout plans for this body type involves a strategic approach to stimulate muscle growth and enhance overall fitness.

1. **Strength Training:**

   - Focus on compound exercises that engage multiple muscle groups, such as squats, deadlifts, and bench presses.

   - Use progressive overload to gradually increase resistance and stimulate muscle growth.

   - Incorporate a mix of free weights and resistance training machines to target different muscle groups.

2. **Frequency and Volume:**

   - Perform weight training sessions three to four times a week to allow for sufficient recovery.

   - Include moderate to high rep ranges (8-12 repetitions) to promote hypertrophy.

3. **Nutrition:**

   - Consume a calorie surplus to support muscle growth.

   - Prioritize protein intake to provide essential amino acids for muscle repair and development.

   - Include a balance of carbohydrates and healthy fats to support overall energy needs.

Customizing Workout Plans for Mesomorphs

Mesomorphs often find it easier to build muscle and maintain a well-defined physique. Customizing workout plans for this body type aims to enhance muscular development while maintaining overall fitness.

1. **Balanced Training:**

   - Incorporate a combination of strength training, cardiovascular exercises, and flexibility training.

   - Emphasize compound movements alongside isolation exercises for targeted muscle development.

   - Include a mix of resistance training and bodyweight exercises for versatility.

2. **Variety and Challenge:**

   - Introduce different workout modalities to prevent monotony and keep the body challenged.

   - Experiment with various workout styles, such as HIIT (High-Intensity Interval Training) and circuit training.

   - Periodically adjust training intensity and volume to avoid plateaus.

3. **Maintaining Muscle Mass:**

   - Engage in regular strength training to preserve muscle mass.

   - Pay attention to overall calorie intake, ensuring it aligns with fitness goals.

   - Include protein-rich foods to support muscle repair and recovery.

Customizing Workout Plans for Endomorphs

Endomorphs may face challenges related to weight management and fat loss. Customizing workout plans for this body type focuses on metabolic conditioning and a balanced approach to achieve overall fitness.

1. **Cardiovascular Exercise:**

   - Incorporate regular cardiovascular exercises to boost metabolism and aid in fat loss.

   - Include activities such as running, cycling, and swimming for effective calorie burning.

   - Experiment with interval training to enhance fat oxidation.

2. **Strength Training for Fat Loss:**

   - Prioritize full-body strength training exercises to stimulate muscle growth and boost metabolism.

   - Integrate circuit training with minimal rest between exercises for an added calorie burn.

   - Include resistance training to maintain and build lean muscle mass.

3. **Nutritional Considerations:**

   - Adopt a well-balanced diet with a slight calorie deficit for gradual fat loss.

   - Focus on whole, nutrient-dense foods to support overall health.

   - Pay attention to portion control and mindful eating habits.

Inclusivity in Fitness: Beyond Body Types

While recognizing body types provides valuable insights into individualized fitness approaches, it is essential to emphasize inclusivity beyond these categories. Every individual has unique strengths, limitations, and preferences that go beyond a standardized classification. Customizing workout plans should consider factors such as:

1. **Individual Goals:**

   - Whether the goal is weight loss, muscle gain, flexibility improvement, or overall well-being, the workout plan should align with individual objectives.

2. **Physical Health Conditions:**

   - Individuals with pre-existing health conditions or injuries may require modifications to accommodate their specific needs.

   - Consultation with healthcare professionals or fitness experts is crucial for safe and effective exercise programming.

3. **Mental and Emotional Well-being:**

   - Incorporating activities that promote mental and emotional well-being, such as yoga, meditation, or dance, contributes to a holistic fitness experience.

4. **Lifestyle and Preferences:**

- Consideration of lifestyle factors, time constraints, and personal preferences ensures that the workout plan is sustainable and enjoyable.

Adapting Fitness Plans Over Time

Fitness is a dynamic journey, and individuals may experience changes in their bodies, goals, and preferences over time. Adapting workout plans to align with evolving needs ensures continued progress and engagement.

1. **Periodization:**

   - Implementing periodization involves dividing training cycles into different phases, each with specific objectives (e.g., strength, hypertrophy, endurance).

   - Periodic changes in intensity, volume, and exercise selection prevent plateaus and support long-term progress.

2. **Skill Development:**

   - Incorporating new activities or skills, such as learning a new sport or participating in group classes, adds variety and maintains interest in fitness.

3. **Listen to Your Body:**

   - Paying attention to signals from the body, including fatigue, soreness, and recovery, allows for adjustments in training intensity and frequency.

Conclusion

In conclusion, the concept of "Fitness for Every Body Type" emphasizes the importance of customizing workout plans based on individual needs and preferences. Recognizing and understanding body types, such as ectomorph, mesomorph, and endomorph, provides a starting point for tailoring exercise routines. However, true inclusivity in fitness goes beyond body classifications, considering individual goals, health conditions, mental well-being, and lifestyle preferences. The dynamic nature of fitness requires ongoing adaptation, with periodic changes to training approaches and the incorporation of new activities. By embracing a personalized and inclusive approach to fitness, individuals can embark on a journey

 that not only enhances physical health but also celebrates the diversity of human bodies and fosters a positive and empowering relationship with exercise.

Chapter 9:

Embracing Mental Wellness

- Strategies for managing stress, anxiety, and fostering mental resilience

Introduction

In the fast-paced and demanding world we live in, the importance of mental wellness cannot be overstated. The pursuit of a balanced and resilient mind is essential for navigating the challenges of daily life. This essay explores the significance of embracing mental wellness, providing insights into effective strategies for managing stress, anxiety, and fostering mental resilience. By understanding the interconnected nature of mental health and adopting proactive measures, individuals can cultivate a resilient mindset that contributes to overall well-being.

Understanding Mental Wellness

Mental wellness encompasses a state of emotional, psychological, and social well-being. It involves the ability to manage stress, cope with life's challenges, and maintain a positive outlook. While mental health focuses on diagnosable conditions, mental wellness extends beyond the absence of mental illness, emphasizing proactive measures to promote a thriving and resilient mind.

The Impact of Stress and Anxiety on Mental Health

Stress and anxiety are pervasive aspects of modern life, affecting individuals across various demographics. Chronic stress and anxiety not only contribute to mental health disorders but also influence physical health, leading to conditions such as cardiovascular disease, compromised immune function, and digestive issues. Recognizing the signs and understanding the impact of stress and anxiety on mental wellness is a crucial first step in fostering resilience.

Strategies for Managing Stress

1. **Mindfulness and Meditation:**

- Mindfulness practices, including meditation and deep-breathing exercises, promote awareness of the present moment.

- Regular mindfulness sessions help reduce stress by calming the mind, improving focus, and fostering a sense of inner peace.

2. **Physical Activity:**

- Regular exercise is a powerful stress reliever, promoting the release of endorphins, the body's natural mood elevators.

- Engaging in activities such as walking, jogging, yoga, or dancing contributes to both physical and mental well-being.

3. **Time Management:**

- Efficient time management minimizes feelings of overwhelm and helps individuals prioritize tasks.

- Breaking down larger tasks into smaller, manageable steps enhances productivity and reduces stress.

4. **Healthy Lifestyle Choices:**

- Adequate sleep, a balanced diet, and hydration play crucial roles in managing stress.

- Limiting caffeine and sugar intake, and prioritizing nutritious foods contribute to overall well-being.

5. **Social Connections:**

- Building and maintaining strong social connections provide a support system during challenging times.

- Sharing concerns with friends or family fosters a sense of connection and emotional support.

Strategies for Managing Anxiety

1. **Cognitive Behavioral Therapy (CBT):**

   - CBT is an evidence-based therapeutic approach that helps individuals identify and change negative thought patterns.

   - Working with a mental health professional trained in CBT can be effective in managing anxiety.

2. **Deep Breathing Exercises:**

   - Controlled breathing techniques, such as diaphragmatic breathing, activate the body's relaxation response and reduce anxiety.

   - Practicing deep breathing regularly enhances emotional regulation.

3. **Progressive Muscle Relaxation (PMR):**

   - PMR involves tensing and then gradually relaxing different muscle groups, promoting physical and mental relaxation.

   - Regular practice helps release tension and reduce overall anxiety levels.

4. **Mind-Body Practices:**

   - Mind-body practices, such as tai chi and qigong, integrate movement, breath control, and meditation to promote relaxation.

   - These practices contribute to a holistic approach to managing anxiety.

5. **Journaling:**

   - Keeping a journal allows individuals to express and process their thoughts and emotions.

   - Identifying triggers and patterns through journaling helps develop self-awareness and coping strategies.

Fostering Mental Resilience

1. **Positive Self-Talk:**

   - Cultivating a positive internal dialogue helps build mental resilience.

   - Challenging negative thoughts and reframing them in a more positive light contributes to a resilient mindset.

2. **Adaptability and Flexibility:**

   - Embracing change and developing adaptability foster mental resilience.

   - Viewing challenges as opportunities for growth rather than insurmountable obstacles enhances resilience.

3. **Seeking Support:**

   - Reaching out for professional help or confiding in friends and family strengthens resilience.

   - Recognizing the importance of seeking support during challenging times is a sign of emotional intelligence.

4. **Mindfulness-Based Stress Reduction (MBSR):**

- MBSR programs combine mindfulness meditation and yoga to reduce stress and enhance resilience.

- Participating in MBSR courses provides practical tools for integrating mindfulness into daily life.

5. **Gratitude Practices:**

- Regularly expressing gratitude has been linked to improved mental well-being.

- Keeping a gratitude journal or simply reflecting on positive aspects of life fosters a resilient perspective.

6. **Setting Realistic Goals:**

- Establishing achievable and realistic goals promotes a sense of accomplishment and resilience.

- Breaking down larger goals into smaller, manageable steps ensures progress and minimizes feelings of overwhelm.

7. **Emotional Regulation:**

- Developing skills for emotional regulation involves recognizing and managing emotions effectively.

- Techniques such as deep breathing, mindfulness, and reframing contribute to emotional resilience.

The Role of Professional Support

In some cases, managing stress, anxiety, and fostering mental resilience may require professional intervention. Mental health professionals, including psychologists, counselors, and psychiatrists, offer specialized expertise and support. Seeking professional help is a proactive step towards building mental resilience and maintaining optimal mental wellness.

Creating a Holistic Approach to Mental Wellness

A holistic approach to mental wellness recognizes the interconnectedness of various aspects of life and emphasizes the integration of physical, emotional, and social well-being.

1. **Holistic Nutrition:**

   - A well-balanced diet that includes nutrient-dense foods contributes to both physical and mental health.

   - Nutrients such as omega-3 fatty acids, vitamins, and minerals play vital roles in brain function and emotional well-being.

2. **Sleep Hygiene:**

   - Prioritizing healthy sleep patterns is essential for cognitive function and emotional regulation.

   - Creating a consistent sleep routine and optimizing sleep environment contribute to overall mental wellness.

3. **Mindful Technology Use:**

   - Managing screen time and practicing mindful technology use promote mental well-being.

   - Unplugging from digital devices during designated periods enhances present-moment awareness.

4. **Nature and Outdoor Activities:**

- Spending time in nature and engaging in outdoor activities have proven mental health benefits.

- Connecting with the natural environment contributes to stress reduction and improved mood.

5. **Educational Resources:**

- Accessing educational resources on mental health topics enhances understanding and promotes self-awareness.

- Books, articles, podcasts, and online courses provide valuable insights into managing stress and anxiety.

Cultivating a Culture of Mental Wellness

Beyond individual efforts, creating a culture of mental wellness involves societal and organizational changes that prioritize mental health.

1. **Reducing Stigma:**

- Destigmatizing mental health encourages open conversations and seeking help without fear of judgment.

- Encouraging workplace and community initiatives that promote mental wellness contributes to stigma reduction.

2. **Workplace Well-being Programs:**

- Implementing well-being programs in workplaces fosters a supportive environment.

- Providing resources, workshops, and mental health days contribute to a culture of mental wellness.

3. **School-Based Mental Health Education:**

   - Integrating mental health education

 into school curriculums raises awareness and equips students with coping skills.

   - Early education on stress management and emotional regulation lays the foundation for lifelong mental wellness.

4. **Community Support Networks:**

   - Developing community-based mental health support networks creates a sense of belonging and solidarity.

   - Community initiatives, such as support groups and mental health awareness campaigns, promote collective well-being.

Conclusion

In conclusion, embracing mental wellness involves a multifaceted approach that addresses stress, anxiety, and fosters mental resilience. Strategies for managing stress and anxiety encompass mindfulness practices, physical activity, time management, and healthy lifestyle choices. Fostering mental resilience involves positive self-talk, adaptability, seeking support, mindfulness-based stress reduction, gratitude practices, and setting realistic goals. Professional support plays a crucial role in cases where additional.intervention is necessary.

The holistic approach to mental wellness extends beyond individual efforts to create a culture that prioritizes mental health. Reducing stigma, implementing workplace well-being programs, integrating mental health education in schools, and fostering community support networks contribute to a comprehensive approach to mental wellness. By understanding the interconnected nature of mental health and adopting proactive strategies, individuals, communities, and organizations can create an environment that embraces mental wellness as an integral component of overall well-being.

Chapter 10:

The Role of Sleep in Transformative Wellness

- Highlighting the significance of quality sleep in overall health

Introduction

In the pursuit of optimal well-being, the role of sleep often takes a backseat as individuals navigate demanding schedules and prioritize various aspects of their lives. However, the significance of quality sleep in transformative wellness cannot be overstated. Sleep is a fundamental biological process that plays a crucial role in physical health, mental well-being, cognitive function, and emotional balance. This essay explores the multifaceted impact of sleep on overall health, emphasizing its transformative power in enhancing the quality of life.

Understanding the Sleep Cycle

Sleep is a complex and dynamic process that occurs in cycles, each consisting of different stages. The sleep cycle comprises two main phases: non-rapid eye movement (NREM) sleep and rapid eye movement (REM) sleep.

1. **NREM Sleep:**

   - NREM sleep is divided into three stages: N1, N2, and N3.

   - N1 is the transitional phase between wakefulness and sleep.

   - N2 is a light sleep stage where the body prepares for deeper sleep.

   - N3, also known as slow-wave sleep, is a deep sleep stage crucial for physical restoration and growth.

2. **REM Sleep:**

   - REM sleep is characterized by rapid eye movements, vivid dreaming, and heightened brain activity.

   - REM sleep is essential for cognitive function, memory consolidation, and emotional processing.

A complete sleep cycle typically lasts about 90 to 110 minutes, and individuals go through multiple cycles during a night of sleep.

The Impact of Quality Sleep on Physical Health

1. **Immune Function:**

   - Quality sleep is closely linked to immune function.

   - During deep sleep stages, the body produces cytokines, proteins that help regulate the immune system and defend against infections.

2. **Cardiovascular Health:**

   - Chronic sleep deprivation is associated with an increased risk of cardiovascular issues, including hypertension and heart disease.

   - Quality sleep supports cardiovascular health by regulating blood pressure and reducing stress on the heart.

3. **Metabolic Health:**

   - Sleep influences metabolic processes, including glucose regulation and insulin sensitivity.

   - Lack of sleep has been linked to an increased risk of obesity and type 2 diabetes.

4. **Hormonal Balance:**

   - Sleep plays a vital role in regulating hormones that affect appetite and metabolism.

   - Disruptions in sleep patterns can lead to imbalances in hormones like leptin and ghrelin, contributing to weight gain.

5. **Muscle Repair and Growth:**

   - Deep sleep stages support muscle repair, growth, and recovery.

   - During slow-wave sleep, the body releases growth hormone, facilitating tissue repair and strengthening.

The Cognitive and Emotional Benefits of Quality Sleep

1. **Memory Consolidation:**

   - REM sleep is crucial for memory consolidation and learning.

   - The brain processes and consolidates information acquired during wakefulness, contributing to improved cognitive function.

2. **Problem-Solving and Creativity:**

   - Quality sleep enhances problem-solving skills and creativity.

   - The brain's ability to make connections and find innovative solutions is optimized during well-rested periods.

3. **Mood Regulation:**

   - Sleep has a profound impact on emotional well-being and mood regulation.

- Adequate sleep supports emotional resilience and helps manage stress, anxiety, and irritability.

4. **Stress Reduction:**

   - Sleep acts as a natural stress regulator.

   - Deep sleep stages promote the release of stress hormones, helping individuals cope with daily challenges more effectively.

The Relationship Between Sleep and Mental Health

1. **Sleep and Mental Health Disorders:**

   - Sleep disturbances are common symptoms of mental health disorders, including depression, anxiety, and bipolar disorder.

   - Addressing sleep issues can be a key component in managing and improving mental health.

2. **Sleep and Cognitive Function:**

   - Chronic sleep deprivation negatively impacts cognitive function, leading to impaired attention, memory, and decision-making.

   - Quality sleep supports cognitive processes, enhancing overall mental acuity.

3. **Sleep and Emotional Regulation:**

   - Sleep plays a crucial role in emotional regulation and resilience.

   - Lack of sleep can contribute to mood swings, heightened emotional reactivity, and increased vulnerability to stressors.

The Importance of Sleep Hygiene

Optimizing the quality of sleep involves adopting healthy sleep hygiene practices. These practices contribute to a conducive sleep environment and promote restful sleep.

1. **Consistent Sleep Schedule:**

   - Going to bed and waking up at the same time every day helps regulate the body's internal clock.

   - Consistency reinforces the circadian rhythm, promoting better sleep quality.

2. **Create a Comfortable Sleep Environment:**

   - Ensure the bedroom is dark, quiet, and cool for optimal sleep.

   - Investing in a comfortable mattress and pillows enhances overall sleep comfort.

3. **Limit Exposure to Screens Before Bed:**

   - The blue light emitted from screens can interfere with melatonin production, disrupting the sleep-wake cycle.

   - Limiting screen time at least an hour before bedtime promotes better sleep quality.

4. **Mindful Relaxation Techniques:**

   - Engaging in relaxation techniques, such as deep breathing, meditation, or progressive muscle relaxation, helps prepare the body for sleep.

- Mindfulness practices promote a calm and relaxed state conducive to restful sleep.

5. **Avoid Stimulants Before Bed:**

   - Limiting caffeine and nicotine intake in the hours leading up to bedtime supports a smoother transition into sleep.

   - Stimulants can interfere with the body's ability to relax and enter restorative sleep.

Addressing Sleep Disorders

While adopting healthy sleep hygiene practices can significantly improve sleep quality, individuals experiencing persistent sleep issues should seek professional evaluation. Sleep disorders, such as insomnia, sleep apnea, and restless legs syndrome, require specialized diagnosis and treatment.

1. **Insomnia:**

   - Insomnia involves difficulty falling asleep or staying asleep, leading to impaired daytime functioning.

   - Cognitive-behavioral therapy for insomnia (CBT-I) is a highly effective non-pharmacological treatment.

2. **Sleep Apnea:**

   - Sleep apnea is characterized by brief interruptions in breathing during sleep.

   - Continuous positive airway pressure (CPAP) therapy is a common treatment for sleep apnea.

3. **Restless Legs Syndrome (RLS):**

   - RLS causes an uncontrollable urge to move the legs, often accompanied by discomfort.

   - Medications and lifestyle modifications can help manage symptoms of RLS.

The Transformative Power of Prioritizing Sleep

1. **Enhanced Productivity and Performance:**

   - Quality sleep enhances cognitive function, concentration, and problem-solving skills.

   - Well-rested individuals are more productive and perform better in both personal and professional pursuits.

2. **Improved Physical Health:**

   - Prioritizing sleep contributes to overall physical health, reducing the risk of chronic diseases and promoting longevity.

   - The body's ability to recover and repair is optimized during restful sleep.

3. **Emotional Resilience and Well-being:**

   - Quality sleep supports emotional resilience, reducing vulnerability to stressors and promoting a positive outlook.

   - Emotional well-being is closely linked to consistent and restorative sleep.

4. **Optimized Cognitive Function:**

- Adequate sleep is vital for optimal cognitive function, memory consolidation, and creative thinking.

   - The transformative power of sleep extends

to improved decision-making and problem-solving abilities.

5. **Enhanced Immune Function:**

   - Quality sleep strengthens the immune system, contributing to better overall health.

   - The body's ability to defend against infections and illnesses is optimized during restorative sleep.

Conclusion

In conclusion, the role of sleep in transformative wellness is profound and far-reaching. Quality sleep is not merely a passive state of rest; it is an active and dynamic process that contributes to physical health, mental well-being, cognitive function, and emotional balance. Recognizing the significance of sleep and prioritizing healthy sleep hygiene practices are essential steps toward achieving transformative wellness.

Individuals, communities, and organizations can contribute to a culture that values and prioritizes sleep as a cornerstone of well-being. By understanding the intricate relationship between sleep and overall health, individuals can embark on a journey that embraces the transformative power of quality sleep, unlocking its potential to enhance the quality of life and promote lasting wellness.

Chapter 11:

Balancing Act: Juggling Fitness, Work, and Life

- Tips for integrating wellness practices into a busy lifestyle

Introduction

In the hustle and bustle of modern life, finding a balance between fitness, work, and personal life can be a challenging endeavor. The demands of a busy schedule often lead individuals to neglect their well-being, both physically and mentally. This essay explores the importance of striking a balance between fitness, work, and life and provides practical tips for integrating wellness practices into a hectic lifestyle. By adopting a holistic approach and implementing manageable strategies, individuals can navigate the delicate balance between their professional responsibilities and personal health, ultimately enhancing overall well-being.

The Significance of Balance in Modern Life

1. **Physical Well-being:**

   - Regular physical activity contributes to physical health, reducing the risk of chronic diseases and promoting longevity.

   - Neglecting fitness can lead to sedentary lifestyles, contributing to issues such as obesity, cardiovascular diseases, and musculoskeletal problems.

2. **Mental Health:**

   - The demands of work and daily life can take a toll on mental health.

   - Engaging in wellness practices, including exercise and stress management, fosters mental resilience and emotional well-being.

3. **Work Productivity:**

   - Balancing fitness and work enhances productivity.

   - Physical activity has been linked to improved cognitive function, concentration, and creativity, positively impacting work performance.

4. **Quality of Life:**

   - Achieving balance contributes to an overall higher quality of life.

   - Integrating wellness practices enhances energy levels, mood, and the ability to enjoy personal and professional pursuits.

Practical Tips for Balancing Fitness, Work, and Life

1. Prioritize and Schedule

a. **Identify Priorities:**

   - Evaluate your core values and priorities in both professional and personal realms.

   - Recognize the importance of health and wellness as a fundamental aspect of a fulfilling life.

b. **Create a Schedule:**

- Develop a realistic and structured daily schedule that accommodates work, fitness, and personal time.

- Allocate specific time blocks for exercise, work tasks, and relaxation.

c. **Set Realistic Goals:**

- Establish achievable fitness and work goals that align with your overall priorities.

- Break down larger goals into smaller, manageable tasks for a sense of accomplishment.

2. Efficient Time Management

a. **Batch Tasks:**

- Group similar tasks together to streamline efficiency.

- This allows for focused work periods, freeing up time for fitness and personal activities.

b. **Limit Multitasking:**

- While multitasking may seem productive, it can lead to decreased efficiency and increased stress.

- Focus on one task at a time to enhance concentration and effectiveness.

c. **Use Breaks Wisely:**

- Incorporate short breaks during work hours for physical activity or mindfulness exercises.

- These breaks can boost energy levels and overall well-being.

3. Embrace Flexible Fitness Options

a. **Home Workouts:**

- Explore home workout options, such as online fitness classes or mobile apps.

- This provides flexibility and eliminates the need for commuting to a gym.

b. **Short, Intense Workouts:**

- Opt for high-intensity interval training (HIIT) or shorter workouts that deliver effective results in less time.

- This is particularly beneficial for those with tight schedules.

c. **Incorporate Activity into Daily Routine:**

- Integrate physical activity into your daily routine, such as walking or cycling to work, taking the stairs, or scheduling walking meetings.

4. Foster a Supportive Work Environment

a. **Encourage Workplace Wellness:**

- Advocate for workplace wellness initiatives that support employee well-being.

- This may include flexible schedules, onsite fitness facilities, or wellness programs.

b. **Establish Boundaries:**

- Set clear boundaries between work and personal time.

- Encourage colleagues to respect these boundaries, promoting a healthier work-life balance.

5. Stress Management and Mindfulness

a. **Practice Mindfulness:**

- Incorporate mindfulness practices, such as meditation or deep-breathing exercises, into your daily routine.

- These practices can help manage stress and improve focus.

b. **Effective Stress Coping Strategies:**

- Identify effective stress coping mechanisms that work for you, such as journaling, hobbies, or spending time in nature.

- Implement these strategies during busy periods to maintain mental well-being.

6. Optimize Sleep

a. **Establish a Sleep Routine:**

- Prioritize sleep by establishing a consistent sleep routine.

- Create a calming bedtime routine and ensure a comfortable sleep environment.

b. **Limit Screen Time Before Bed:**

- Reduce exposure to screens at least an hour before bedtime to promote better sleep quality.

- Blue light emitted by screens can interfere with the body's production of melatonin, a sleep-inducing hormone.

c. **Quality Over Quantity:**

- Focus on the quality of sleep rather than sheer hours.

- Aim for restful and uninterrupted sleep to support overall well-being.

7. Learn to Say No

a. **Set Boundaries:**

- Recognize your limitations and set boundaries to prevent overcommitting.

- Learning to say no when necessary is crucial for maintaining balance.

b. **Prioritize Self-Care:**

- Prioritize self-care without feeling guilty.

- Taking time for yourself is essential for recharging and maintaining a sustainable balance.

8. Reflect and Adjust

a. **Regular Reflection:**

   - Reflect on your schedule and well-being regularly.

   - Assess what is working and what needs adjustment.

b. **Adaptability:**

   - Be adaptable and open to adjusting your routine as circumstances change.

   - Life is dynamic, and flexibility is key to maintaining balance.

9. Invest in Personal Development

a. **Continuous Learning:**

   - Invest time in continuous learning and personal development.

   - Expanding your skills and knowledge can contribute to career advancement and personal fulfillment.

b. **Explore Interests:**

   - Dedicate time to explore personal interests and hobbies

   - Engaging in activities you love contributes to a more fulfilling and balanced life.

10. Seek Professional Guidance

a. **Consult with Experts:**

- Consult with fitness professionals or health experts to design a personalized fitness plan.

- Seeking advice from professionals ensures a tailored approach that aligns with individual needs.

b. **Career Counseling:**

- Consider career counseling or coaching to align your professional path with personal goals.

- Professional guidance can provide clarity and support in achieving a fulfilling career.

Conclusion

In conclusion, the balancing act of juggling fitness, work, and life is a dynamic and ongoing process that requires intentional effort and mindfulness. By prioritizing well-being, adopting efficient time management strategies, and incorporating flexible fitness options, individuals can strike a balance that promotes physical and mental health. Fostering a supportive work environment, practicing stress management and mindfulness, and optimizing sleep contribute to a holistic approach to well-being.

The key lies in recognizing the interconnectedness of different aspects of life and acknowledging the importance of balance. Implementing these practical tips empowers individuals to navigate their busy lives with greater ease, fostering a sense of fulfillment, resilience, and transformative well-being. Ultimately, the journey towards balance is a personal one, and by embracing intentional choices and lifestyle adjustments, individuals can achieve a harmonious integration of fitness, work, and life.

Chapter 12:

Holistic Approaches to Weight Management

- Exploring sustainable methods for achieving and maintaining a healthy weight

Holistic Approaches to Weight Management: Nurturing Well-Being from Within

Introduction:

In a world inundated with fad diets, quick fixes, and magic pills promising rapid weight loss, the importance of adopting a holistic approach to weight management cannot be overstated. Rather than focusing solely on shedding pounds, a holistic perspective recognizes the interconnectedness of physical, mental, and emotional well-being. This comprehensive view seeks sustainable methods for achieving and maintaining a healthy weight that goes beyond mere calorie counting. In this exploration, we will delve into the multifaceted nature of holistic weight management, emphasizing lifestyle choices, nutrition, physical activity, and the psychological aspects that contribute to overall well-being.

1. Understanding Holistic Weight Management:

At its core, holistic weight management is about recognizing that the body is a complex system where various factors contribute to overall health. Instead of isolating weight loss as a goal, this approach emphasizes creating a balance in different aspects of life to foster well-being. It encompasses physical health, mental and emotional stability, social connections, and environmental factors. By addressing these interrelated components, individuals can embark on a journey towards sustainable weight management.

2. Lifestyle Choices:

One of the fundamental pillars of holistic weight management lies in adopting a healthy lifestyle. This involves cultivating habits that promote overall well-being, including sufficient sleep, stress management, and the avoidance of harmful substances. Sleep, in particular, plays a crucial role in regulating hormones related to hunger and satiety. Chronic stress, on the other hand, can lead to emotional eating and disrupted metabolic processes. By fostering a balanced lifestyle, individuals set a solid foundation for achieving and maintaining a healthy weight.

3. Nutrition as Nourishment:

Holistic weight management places a significant emphasis on nutrition, viewing food not just as a source of calories but as a means of nourishment for the body and mind. Instead of subscribing to restrictive diets, the focus is on adopting a balanced and sustainable eating pattern. This might include incorporating a variety of whole foods, emphasizing fruits, vegetables, lean proteins, and whole grains. By nourishing the body with essential nutrients, individuals support their overall health and create a sustainable approach to weight management.

4. Physical Activity:

The role of physical activity in holistic weight management cannot be overstated. Exercise not only contributes to calorie expenditure but also has a profound impact on mental health. It releases endorphins, the body's natural mood enhancers, and supports overall well-being. A holistic approach to physical activity involves finding activities that are enjoyable and sustainable rather than focusing solely on rigorous workouts. This could be anything from walking and cycling to yoga and dance. By integrating movement into daily life, individuals not only contribute to weight management but also enhance their overall quality of life.

5. Psychological Aspects:

The psychological aspects of weight management are often underestimated. Holistic approaches recognize the intricate relationship between emotions, mindset, and eating behaviors. Emotional eating, for instance, is a common response to stress, sadness, or boredom. By addressing the root causes of such behaviors, individuals can develop healthier coping mechanisms. Mindful eating, meditation, and cognitive-behavioral strategies are integral components of holistic weight management, fostering a positive relationship with food and promoting long-term success.

6. Hormonal Balance:

The intricate interplay of hormones within the body plays a crucial role in weight management. Holistic approaches consider hormonal balance as a key factor, acknowledging that imbalances can affect metabolism, appetite, and energy expenditure. Factors such as adequate sleep, stress management, and proper nutrition contribute to hormonal equilibrium. By understanding and addressing hormonal influences, individuals can optimize their body's natural processes, making weight management more effective and sustainable.

7. Social Support and Community:

Weight management is not a solitary endeavor. Holistic approaches recognize the importance of social connections and community support. Engaging with others who share similar health goals can provide motivation, accountability, and a sense of belonging. Whether through group exercise classes, online communities, or support from friends and family, the social dimension of holistic weight management reinforces the idea that well-being is a collective effort.

8. Environmental Considerations:

The environment in which individuals live can significantly impact their ability to maintain a healthy weight. Holistic approaches take into account factors such as access to nutritious food, opportunities for physical activity, and the influence of the built environment. Creating environments that support healthy choices, such as walkable neighborhoods and access to fresh produce, can contribute to the success of weight management initiatives.

9. Holistic Weight Management for Long-Term Success:

The essence of holistic weight management lies in its focus on long-term well-being rather than quick fixes. Sustainable weight management is not about following a rigid plan for a short period but rather involves making gradual, lasting changes to one's lifestyle. This requires patience, self-compassion, and a commitment to ongoing self-improvement. Holistic approaches acknowledge that setbacks are a natural part of the journey and encourage individuals to learn from them rather than viewing them as failures.

10. Challenges and Criticisms:

While holistic approaches to weight management offer a comprehensive and sustainable perspective, they are not without challenges and criticisms. Some argue that the individualized nature of holistic strategies makes it difficult to create standardized interventions. Additionally, the emphasis on addressing multiple aspects of life may seem overwhelming for some individuals, leading to a perception of complexity. It's essential to recognize these challenges and work towards creating accessible and supportive frameworks for holistic weight management.

Conclusion:

In conclusion, holistic approaches to weight management provide a nuanced and sustainable perspective on achieving and maintaining a healthy weight. By recognizing the interconnectedness of physical, mental, and emotional well-being, individuals can embark on a journey that goes beyond calorie counting and restrictive diets. Lifestyle choices, nutrition, physical activity, psychological aspects, hormonal balance, social support, and environmental considerations all play integral roles in the holistic approach. The emphasis on long-term well-being, self-compassion, and gradual changes sets the foundation for a healthier and more fulfilling life. As we continue to explore and refine holistic strategies, we move towards a future where weight management is not just about numbers on a scale but a holistic expression of a well-nurtured, vibrant life.

Chapter 13:

Superfoods and Nutritional Powerhouses

- Identifying nutrient-rich foods for optimal health and vitality

Superfoods and Nutritional Powerhouses: Unveiling the Secrets of Nature's Bounty for Optimal Health and Vitality

Introduction:

In the quest for optimal health and vitality, the concept of "superfoods" has gained prominence. These nutrient-rich foods are often hailed for their exceptional health benefits and high concentration of vitamins, minerals, antioxidants, and other essential nutrients. In this exploration, we will delve into the world of superfoods, examining what makes them nutritional powerhouses, their impact on overall health, and how incorporating them into our diets can contribute to a lifestyle that nurtures both the body and mind.

1. Defining Superfoods:

The term "superfood" is not a scientific classification, but rather a marketing buzzword used to describe foods that are exceptionally nutrient-dense and believed to confer health benefits. These foods are typically rich in antioxidants, vitamins, minerals, and other bioactive compounds. While there is no official list of superfoods, many share common characteristics such as being dense in nutrients, low in calories, and offering a range of health-promoting properties.

2. Nutrient-Rich Powerhouses:

What sets superfoods apart is their ability to pack a powerful nutritional punch in relatively small servings. From berries like blueberries and acai to leafy greens like kale and spinach, these foods are brimming with essential nutrients. They provide a concentrated source of vitamins (such as vitamin C, K, and various B vitamins), minerals (including iron, potassium, and magnesium), and phytochemicals with antioxidant properties.

3. Antioxidants and Free Radicals:

One of the key attributes of many superfoods is their high antioxidant content. Antioxidants play a crucial role in neutralizing free radicals in the body. Free radicals are unstable molecules that can damage cells and contribute to aging and various diseases. By consuming foods rich in antioxidants, individuals can support their bodies in combating oxidative stress and promoting overall well-being.

4. Popular Superfoods:

Numerous foods have been designated as superfoods, each offering a unique set of nutrients and health benefits. Berries, such as blueberries, strawberries, and goji berries, are celebrated for their antioxidant content. Leafy greens like kale and spinach are powerhouse vegetables packed with vitamins and minerals. Fatty fish, such as salmon and mackerel, provide omega-3 fatty acids, known for their heart-healthy properties. Other examples include nuts and seeds, quinoa, turmeric, and green tea. Exploring these superfoods allows individuals to diversify their nutrient intake and harness a broad spectrum of health benefits.

5. Incorporating Superfoods into the Diet:

While the idea of superfoods is appealing, it's crucial to approach them as part of a balanced and varied diet. No single food can provide all the nutrients the body needs for optimal health. Instead, the key lies in incorporating a variety of nutrient-dense foods into one's daily meals. This could involve adding berries to breakfast, including leafy greens in salads, incorporating fatty fish into dinners, and snacking on nuts and seeds. By diversifying the diet with superfoods, individuals can enhance their overall nutrient intake.

6. Adaptogens and Functional Foods:

Beyond the traditional superfoods, there's a growing interest in adaptogens and functional foods. Adaptogens are a class of herbs and mushrooms that are believed to help the body adapt to stress and maintain balance. Examples include ashwagandha, rhodiola, and reishi mushrooms. Functional foods are those that provide health benefits beyond basic nutrition. For instance, probiotics found in fermented foods like yogurt and kimchi support gut health. Exploring these categories broadens the spectrum of nutrient-rich options available for those seeking to optimize their health.

7. Superfoods for Specific Health Goals:

Different superfoods offer specific health benefits, making them particularly relevant for individuals with specific health goals. For example, chia seeds and flaxseeds are rich in omega-3 fatty acids and fiber, making them beneficial for heart health and digestive function. Turmeric, with its active compound curcumin, is known for its anti-inflammatory properties. Understanding the unique benefits of each superfood allows individuals to tailor their dietary choices to align with their health objectives.

8. Plant-Based Superfoods:

With the rise of plant-based diets, many superfoods are plant-derived, showcasing the nutritional richness of fruits, vegetables, nuts, and seeds. Plant-based superfoods not only contribute to overall health but also align with sustainability and environmental consciousness. The inclusion of foods like quinoa, lentils, and plant-based protein sources underscores the diverse options available for those choosing plant-centric diets.

9. Challenges and Considerations:

While superfoods offer numerous health benefits, it's essential to approach them with a balanced perspective. Relying solely on specific foods as a shortcut to health may lead to nutritional imbalances. Additionally, the availability and affordability of certain superfoods may pose challenges for some individuals. It's crucial to recognize that a varied and balanced diet, including a range of nutrient-dense foods, is the foundation for optimal health.

10. Beyond Superfoods: Holistic Nutrition:

While superfoods capture attention for their extraordinary nutrient content, holistic nutrition emphasizes the overall quality of one's diet. It considers the synergistic effects of various foods and encourages a mindful and intuitive approach to eating. Instead of focusing solely on individual superfoods, holistic nutrition encourages individuals to consider the broader context of their dietary patterns, including meal timing, food combinations, and the overall balance of macronutrients.

11. Superfoods and Aging:

As individuals age, nutritional needs may change, and incorporating superfoods into the diet can play a role in supporting healthy aging. Foods rich in antioxidants, such as berries and leafy greens, may contribute to cognitive health. Adequate protein intake, including sources like fatty fish, nuts, and seeds, becomes crucial for maintaining muscle mass. Superfoods can be valuable allies in promoting vitality and well-being throughout the aging process.

Conclusion:

In conclusion, superfoods and nutritional powerhouses represent a diverse array of nutrient-dense foods that can significantly contribute to optimal health and vitality. Whether through their antioxidant content, rich vitamin and mineral profiles, or unique health-promoting compounds, these foods offer a multitude of benefits. However, it's important to approach superfoods as part of a well-rounded and balanced diet. The key lies not in relying on a single magical food but in embracing a variety of nutrient-dense options that collectively nourish the body and mind. As we continue to unravel the nutritional secrets of nature's bounty, we embark on a journey towards a holistic and sustainable approach to health and well-being.

Chapter 14:

Incorporating Wellness into Daily Habits

- Practical tips for creating lasting healthy habits

Incorporating Wellness into Daily Habits: A Blueprint for Lasting Health and Vitality

Introduction:

Wellness is not a destination but a journey, and its essence lies in the daily habits that shape our lives. Incorporating wellness into our daily routines is more than a goal; it's a commitment to nurturing our physical, mental, and emotional well-being. In this exploration, we will delve into practical tips and strategies for seamlessly integrating wellness into our daily habits. From mindful eating and regular exercise to stress management and adequate sleep, these habits form the foundation for a life imbued with lasting health and vitality.

1. The Power of Habits:

Habits are the building blocks of our daily lives. They are the routines and behaviors that shape our experiences and, over time, become ingrained into our lifestyles. By understanding the psychology of habit formation, individuals can intentionally cultivate habits that promote wellness. Charles Duhigg's habit loop—cue, routine, reward—provides a framework for understanding how habits work and how to modify or create them effectively.

2. Morning Rituals for a Healthy Start:

The way we start our mornings sets the tone for the rest of the day. Incorporating wellness into the early hours can have a profound impact on our overall well-being. Morning rituals might include practices such as hydration with lemon water, stretching or yoga, and mindful breathing exercises. These rituals not only promote physical health but also create a positive mindset for the day ahead.

3. Mindful Eating:

Eating is a fundamental aspect of daily life, and adopting mindful eating habits can transform our relationship with food. Mindful eating involves paying full attention to the sensory experience of eating, savoring each bite, and recognizing hunger and fullness cues. By slowing down and being present during meals, individuals can develop a healthier attitude toward food, fostering better digestion and overall well-being.

4. Hydration as a Cornerstone:

Staying adequately hydrated is a simple yet powerful habit that contributes to overall wellness. Water is essential for numerous bodily functions, including digestion, nutrient absorption, and temperature regulation. Incorporating hydration into daily habits involves carrying a reusable water bottle, setting reminders, and infusing water with fruits or herbs for added flavor. The benefits of proper hydration extend beyond physical health, influencing mental clarity and energy levels.

5. Regular Exercise for Physical and Mental Fitness:

Exercise is a cornerstone of wellness, offering a myriad of benefits for both physical and mental health. Creating a habit of regular exercise involves finding activities that are enjoyable and sustainable. This might include walking, jogging, cycling, swimming, or engaging in group fitness classes. Consistency is key, and incorporating exercise into daily routines, such as morning or lunchtime workouts, helps establish a lasting habit.

6. Prioritizing Sleep for Restoration:

Quality sleep is foundational to overall well-being, influencing cognitive function, mood, and physical health. Establishing a consistent sleep routine is crucial for creating healthy sleep habits. This includes maintaining a regular sleep schedule, creating a comfortable sleep environment, and adopting pre-sleep relaxation practices. Prioritizing sleep as an essential aspect of daily self-care contributes to enhanced vitality and resilience.

7. Stress Management Techniques:

In the fast-paced modern world, stress management is a vital component of wellness. Developing habits that help mitigate stress can significantly impact both mental and physical health. Practices such as meditation, deep breathing exercises, mindfulness, and hobbies that promote relaxation are effective tools for managing stress. By integrating these techniques into daily routines, individuals build resilience and cultivate a sense of balance.

8. Digital Detox and Mindful Technology Use:

In an era dominated by technology, incorporating wellness into daily habits also involves mindful use of digital devices. Establishing boundaries for screen time, implementing regular digital detox periods, and creating tech-free zones in the home contribute to a healthier relationship with technology. This not only supports mental well-being but also fosters more meaningful connections with the surrounding environment.

9. Cultivating Emotional Well-Being:

Emotional wellness is an integral aspect of overall well-being, and habits that nurture emotional health are essential. This might involve expressing gratitude daily, practicing self-compassion, and maintaining healthy social connections. Journaling, engaging in creative pursuits, and seeking professional support when needed are additional strategies for cultivating emotional resilience.

10. Incorporating Nutrient-Rich Foods:

Nutrition plays a pivotal role in wellness, and incorporating nutrient-rich foods into daily habits is a fundamental step toward optimal health. This involves choosing a variety of whole foods, including fruits, vegetables, lean proteins, whole grains, and healthy fats. Planning and preparing meals ahead of time, mindful grocery shopping, and experimenting with new recipes contribute to a well-rounded and nourishing diet.

11. Building a Supportive Community:

Wellness is not a solitary journey, and building a supportive community reinforces healthy habits. Connecting with like-minded individuals, whether through local fitness groups, online communities, or wellness events, provides encouragement, accountability, and a sense of belonging. Sharing experiences and learning from others contribute to the ongoing evolution of wellness habits.

12. Continuous Learning and Adaptation:

Incorporating wellness into daily habits is a dynamic process that requires continuous learning and adaptation. Staying informed about new research, emerging trends in health and wellness, and personal preferences allows individuals to refine their habits over time. The willingness to adapt and evolve ensures that wellness practices remain relevant and sustainable throughout different phases of life.

13. Creating a Wellness-Focused Environment:

The physical environment significantly influences daily habits. Creating a wellness-focused environment involves organizing spaces to support healthy behaviors. This might include setting up a dedicated workout area at home, having a well-stocked kitchen with nutritious foods, and creating spaces for relaxation and mindfulness. The alignment of the physical environment with wellness goals enhances the likelihood of maintaining healthy habits.

14. Tracking Progress and Celebrating Achievements:

Monitoring progress and celebrating achievements are integral to sustaining wellness habits. Keeping a wellness journal, using tracking apps, or setting specific goals can provide a sense of direction and accomplishment. Recognizing and celebrating milestones, whether they are related to fitness, nutrition, or stress management, reinforces the positive aspects of wellness-focused habits.

15. Overcoming Challenges and Staying Resilient:

In the journey toward incorporating wellness into daily habits, challenges are inevitable. Whether it's facing time constraints, dealing with unexpected stressors, or navigating setbacks, staying resilient is key. Developing a mindset that embraces setbacks as opportunities for learning, seeking support when needed, and maintaining a flexible approach to wellness habits contribute to long-term success.

Conclusion:

In conclusion, incorporating wellness into daily habits is a transformative journey that requires intention, commitment, and adaptability. From mindful eating and regular exercise to stress management and quality sleep, these habits form the mosaic of a life infused with health and vitality. By embracing the power of habits, individuals can weave wellness into the fabric of their daily lives, creating a sustainable foundation for lasting well-being. The key lies not in drastic changes but in the cumulative effect of small, intentional actions that collectively contribute to a life rich in health and vitality.

Chapter 15:

Celebrating Your Transformation

- Reflecting on progress and maintaining long-term well-being

Celebrating Your Transformation: Reflection, Progress, and Long-Term Well-Being

Introduction:

Transformation is a dynamic and ongoing process that extends beyond physical changes. Celebrating your transformation involves not only recognizing the progress you've made but also fostering a mindset that embraces personal growth and long-term well-being. In this exploration, we will delve into the importance of reflection, acknowledging achievements, and establishing sustainable practices to maintain overall health and vitality.

1. Transformation Beyond the Physical:

While physical changes may be the most visible aspects of transformation, celebrating your journey involves acknowledging the mental, emotional, and spiritual shifts that accompany it. This holistic perspective recognizes that well-being encompasses more than just appearance. It involves cultivating resilience, nurturing positive mental health, and fostering a sense of purpose and fulfillment.

2. The Power of Reflection:

Reflection is a powerful tool for personal growth and transformation. Taking time to reflect on your journey allows you to gain insights into the choices you've made, the challenges you've overcome, and the lessons you've learned. Regular reflection promotes self-awareness and a deeper understanding of your values, priorities, and aspirations. This introspective practice lays the foundation for celebrating your transformation with authenticity and gratitude.

3. Acknowledging Progress, Big and Small:

Transformation is a series of incremental steps, and acknowledging both big milestones and small victories is crucial. Whether it's reaching a fitness goal, making healthier food choices, or adopting positive habits, each step contributes to the overall transformation. Celebrating progress reinforces a positive mindset and motivates further growth. Keeping a journal or creating a progress board can serve as visual reminders of achievements, serving as a source of inspiration during challenging times.

4. Cultivating a Positive Mindset:

A positive mindset is a cornerstone of celebrating your transformation. This involves reframing challenges as opportunities for learning and growth. Rather than focusing on perceived shortcomings, cultivating gratitude for the progress made creates a positive narrative around your transformation journey. Mindfulness practices, affirmations, and surrounding yourself with positive influences contribute to a mindset that fosters well-being.

5. Setting Realistic and Sustainable Goals:

Transformation is a journey, not a destination, and setting realistic and sustainable goals is essential for long-term success. Rather than fixating on quick fixes or temporary changes, focus on creating habits and goals that align with your values and can be maintained over time. This might involve breaking down larger goals into smaller, manageable steps and adjusting them as needed based on your evolving priorities.

6. Nurturing Emotional Well-Being:

Celebrating your transformation extends beyond physical health to include emotional well-being. Cultivating emotional intelligence, practicing self-compassion, and seeking support when needed are integral components of this journey. Acknowledging and addressing emotional challenges allows for a more holistic celebration of transformation, fostering resilience and emotional strength.

7. Embracing Flexibility and Adaptability:

Life is dynamic, and transformational journeys often involve unexpected twists and turns. Embracing flexibility and adaptability is crucial for maintaining well-being over the long term. Rather than rigidly adhering to a specific plan, be open to adjusting your goals and habits based on changing circumstances. This adaptability ensures that your transformation remains a sustainable and evolving process.

8. Integrating Joyful Movement:

Physical activity is not only essential for physical health but also contributes to emotional well-being. Celebrate your transformation by integrating joyful movement into your daily life. Whether it's dancing, hiking, practicing yoga, or participating in a team sport, finding activities that bring joy enhances your overall well-being. The enjoyment derived from movement reinforces a positive relationship with exercise, making it a sustainable and fulfilling part of your routine.

9. Mindful Nutrition:

Nourishing your body with mindful nutrition is a celebration of your transformation from the inside out. Instead of restrictive diets, focus on intuitive eating, paying attention to hunger and fullness cues, and savoring the flavors of wholesome foods. This approach not only supports physical health but also fosters a positive and sustainable relationship with food, contributing to long-term well-being.

10. Cultivating Meaningful Connections:

Transformation is often intertwined with personal relationships. Cultivating meaningful connections with others provides a sense of support and community on your journey. Share your achievements with friends or family, or consider joining groups or communities with similar interests and goals. Celebrating your transformation becomes more meaningful when it is shared with those who genuinely appreciate and support your growth.

11. Continuous Learning and Evolution:

A commitment to continuous learning and evolution is fundamental to celebrating your transformation. Stay curious about new ways to enhance your well-being, whether through exploring different forms of exercise, adopting new mindfulness practices, or expanding your knowledge of nutrition. Embracing a growth mindset ensures that your celebration is not a static event but an ongoing and evolving process.

12. Engaging in Purposeful Activities:

Transformation gains depth and meaning when it aligns with your sense of purpose. Engaging in activities that bring a sense of fulfillment and purpose contributes to your overall well-being. This might involve volunteering, pursuing creative passions, or participating in activities that resonate with your values. Celebrating your transformation becomes a holistic experience when it is intertwined with a sense of purpose and contribution to the broader community.

13. Establishing Rituals of Self-Care:

Self-care is a fundamental aspect of celebrating your transformation. Establishing rituals of self-care involves regular practices that nurture your physical, mental, and emotional well-being. This might include taking time for relaxation, pampering yourself with spa-like activities, or simply enjoying moments of solitude. These rituals serve as anchors in your routine, fostering a continuous celebration of your commitment to well-being.

14. Reflecting on Gratitude:

Expressing gratitude for the journey and the support you've received is a powerful way to celebrate your transformation. Reflect on the people, experiences, and opportunities that have contributed to your growth. Gratitude practices, such as keeping a gratitude journal or expressing appreciation to others, enhance your overall well-being and create a positive perspective on your transformational journey.

15. Seeking Professional Guidance:

Celebrating your transformation may also involve seeking professional guidance when needed. Whether it's consulting with a nutritionist, a fitness trainer, or a mental health professional, recognizing when additional support is beneficial is a sign of self-awareness and commitment to your well-being. Professional guidance can provide personalized insights and strategies that complement your transformational journey.

Conclusion:

In conclusion, celebrating your transformation is a multifaceted and ongoing process that extends beyond the physical realm. It involves reflection, acknowledging progress, cultivating a positive mindset, and establishing sustainable practices for long-term well-being. Transformation is not a destination but a continuous journey that embraces personal growth, resilience, and a holistic approach to health and vitality. By integrating these principles into your daily life, you embark on a celebration that unfolds authentically, providing a foundation for lasting well-being and fulfillment.